Speci   *Recovery*

"Kyczy Hawk has done something extraordinary with her
new book, *Yogic Tools for Recovery*. With expert composition,
Kyczy has made it possible to walk the path of recovery from any
addiction by embracing two of the most powerful approaches of
our time: yoga and the Twelve Steps. The manner in which she
presents this material gives access to any person who earnestly
seeks to live one day at a time in that exalted place beyond
addiction. One path to balance and long-term, sustainable
recovery is laid out brilliantly in this wonderful book."

Tommy Rosen, founder of Recovery 2.0

"*Yogic Tools for Recovery* is filled with wisdom and practices
to deepen recovery from any addiction. Kyczy has created an
important resource for the practical application of yoga and
twelve-step program principles. This book will be useful for
anyone who is serious about addiction recovery.'"

R. Nikki Myers, founder of Y12SR: The Yoga of 12-Step Recovery

"Love it! In *Yogic Tools for Recovery,* Kyczy has a wonderful
way of blending the Twelve Steps with yogic philosophy to help
reinvigorate one's recovery. By combining the practice of yoga,
breath work, meditation, and the principles of the Steps, it takes
us to a new level in our recovery process. It rejuvenates the mind,
body, and spirit, so we can see our recovery through a different
lens with greater clarity and a new perspective."

Ron Tannebaum, cofounder InTheRooms.com

"Kyczy Hawk is a true pioneer in the yoga recovery movement, quietly blazing a path for others on a journey of recovery as they discover the healing gifts of yoga at their own pace. In this book, Kyczy offers individuals working a twelve-step program practical, applicable teaching for blending yoga into the healing made available to us in the Twelve Steps. The wisdom that Kyczy, a gifted teacher, shares with individuals in recovery, or those seeking some kind of change in life, emanates from the pages. Exploring this book will likely be one of the most powerful decisions you can make as you explore your options for healing and wholeness."

Jamie Marich, PhD, clinical trauma expert and author of
Trauma and the Twelve Steps and *Dancing Mindfulness*

"*Yogic Tools for Recovery* is an excellent resource for anymore looking to add a physical practice to their spiritual program. Kyczy carefully blends simple yoga poses and holistic yoga philosophy with traditional twelve-step recovery in a unique and inspiring way. This book is a joy."

Gregory S. Pergament, author of *Chi Kung in Recovery*

"Both twelve-step recovery and yoga have been part of my life for many years, so I am delighted to discover *Yogic Tools for Recovery*. Hawk elegantly and compellingly articulates the philosophies and practical application of each, and she provides a thoughtful bridge between yoga—its philosophy, lineage, and language—and the philosophy, literature, and practical tools of twelve-step recovery. *Yogic Tools for Recovery* is the perfect handbook to help us work the Twelve Steps through yoga, while fully honoring the traditions of recovery. Hawk's book will sit next to your mat *and* your Big Book or Basic Text, enabling a truly holistic recovery."

Diane Cameron, registered yoga teacher and author
of *Out of the Woods* and *Never Leave Your Dead*

YOGIC TOOLS FOR RECOVERY

A GUIDE FOR WORKING THE TWELVE STEPS

YOGIC TOOLS
for Recovery

KYCZY HAWK

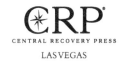

CRP
CENTRAL RECOVERY PRESS
LAS VEGAS

Central Recovery Press (CRP) is committed to publishing exceptional materials addressing addiction treatment, recovery, and behavioral healthcare topics.

For more information, visit www.centralrecoverypress.com.

Publisher: Central Recovery Press
             3321 N. Buffalo Drive
             Las Vegas, NV 89129

22 21 20 19 18 17   1 2 3 4 5

Library of Congress Cataloging-in-Publication Data
Names: Hawk, Kyczy.
Title: Yogic tools for recovery : a guide for working the twelve steps / Kyczy Hawk.
Description: Las Vegas : Central Recovery Press, 2017.
Identifiers: LCCN 2017023598 (print) | LCCN 2017039084 (ebook) | ISBN 9781942094531 (e-book) | ISBN 9781942094524 (paperback)
Subjects: LCSH: Self-actualization (Psychology) | Yoga. | Twelve-step programs. | BISAC: SELF-HELP / Twelve-Step Programs. | HEALTH & FITNESS / Yoga. | BODY, MIND & SPIRIT / Inspiration & Personal Growth. | HEALTH & FITNESS / Exercise.
Classification: LCC BF637.S4 (ebook) | LCC BF637.S4 H39 2017 (print) | DDC 181/.45--dc23
LC record available at https://lccn.loc.gov/2017023598

Photo of Kyczy Hawk by William Hawk. Used with permission.

The Twelve Steps of Narcotics Anonymous. Reprinted by permission of NA World Services, Inc. All rights reserved. The Twelve Steps of NA reprinted for adaptation by permission of A.A. World Services, Inc.

pp. Title, 4, 6, 7–8, 37, 58, 81, 94, 124, 133, 144, 155: *The Yoga Sutras of Patanjali* by Gary Kissiah. Copyright Lilalabs Publishing LLC, 2016; p. 5: © *Twelve Steps and Twelve Traditions,* page 46, is reprinted with permission of A.A. World Services, Inc.; p. 106: © *Alcoholics Anonymous,* pages 76 and 77, is reprinted with permission of A.A. World Services, Inc.; p. 128: Used with permission from Reverend Jaganath Carrera; p. 144: From *The Heart of Yoga* by T. K.V. Desikachar, ©1995. Reprinted by permission of Inner Traditions International and Bear & Company. www.innertraditions.com; p. 167: Excerpt(s) from BHAGAVAD GITA: A NEW TRANSLATION by Stephen Mitchell, copyright ©2000 by Stephen Mitchell. Used by permission of Harmony Books, an imprint of the Crown Publishing Group, a division of Penguin Random House LLC. All rights reserved; p. 167: From *The Teachings of Yogi Bhagan.* Used by permission from the Kundalini Research Institute, www.kriteachings.org.

Every attempt has been made to contact copyright holders. If copyright holders have not been properly acknowledged, please contact us. Central Recovery Press will be happy to rectify the omission in future printings of this book.

Publisher's Note: This book contains general information about yoga, addiction, addiction recovery, and related matters. The information is not medical advice. This book is not an alternative to medical advice from your doctor or other professional healthcare provider. Our books represent the experiences and opinions of their authors only. Every effort has been made to ensure that events, institutions, and statistics presented in our books as facts are accurate and up-to-date. To protect their privacy, the names of some of the people, places, and institutions in this book may have been changed.

Cover and interior design and layout by Sara Streifel, Think Creative Design

"Sorrow which is yet to come
should be avoided."

SUTRA 2.16

Table of Contents

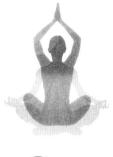

Preface

This is going to be hard. Working the steps is already difficult. Learning a new language is challenging. Incorporating a new perspective into the process will require effort. And, it is all worth it. Nothing compares to the pain of stalling out in your recovery, knowing that there is more to life and not being able to access it. Maybe there are unknown skeletons from the past, wreckage created during recovery, or something impeding you from embracing your beautiful present and future. Recovery may no longer be enjoyable; relapse could be just around the corner.

That is what it was like for me. Unaddressed issues choked me. I floundered in my practiced way of working the program. I did not relapse using drugs or alcohol, but I dove headlong into another addiction. Society loves this addiction, but my mind, body, and spirit did not: I submerged myself in my work.

One of the dangers was that I could have thought I was cured, that I was doing well in my profession so I didn't need the program, maybe I wasn't an alcoholic. I had been living in a bad situation, struggling with my economic circumstances and being a single mom. Excuses and reasons abounded. I was doing a fabulous job at work; I was "successful" and motivated.

I was close enough to my friends in the program and to my sponsor that I heard myself talking this trash. And, that is where relapse starts—with the garbage your addiction-prone mind will tell you. I was terrified and exhausted and out of touch with myself—my feelings, my body, and my soul. I knew I was in trouble. I just didn't know how to get out of it.

Even though I had been in a recovery running group, going to one or two meetings a week and getting together with my sponsor and sponsees, I was dry in all senses of the word. I was empty on the inside; I was clean and sober but not happy, joyous, or free. I was depressed and hollow. I feared the worst, and my terror led me to yoga.

Previously, I had practiced some yoga using videos. I knew some information about the benefits of an integrated body, mind, and spirit that yoga was said to provide. I was curious. Could this help? I was desperate. With reluctance and doubt, I attended my first class at a health food store in 2004. It was difficult. I was tense and inflexible. My body hurt, and I cried. My tears were not from physical pain but from emotional release. I returned again and again. The improvement in my mind, body, and spirit were greater than the discomfort of the practice. There was something magical going on.

The poses, the breath, and the meditation helped me reinhabit my body. While in my fever of overworking, I had neglected my body in the most terrible way. I wasn't sleeping well. I exercised as a type of punishment rather than communion. I didn't eat well or in a nourishing way—gobbling a bagel in the car while I drove to work, heating up packages of frozen vegetables with sauce and eating them at my desk, skipping meals entirely, or binging on late-night pizza while we worked. I even neglected to use the toilet when I needed to, telling myself that I would go after I finished one more thing. I got bruises from banging into desks and doorways and tripped often racing to the copy machine, printer, or someone's office. I was not in my body. Yoga reminded me of that and helped me move back in.

It turned out I had tapped only the tiniest bit of the font of recovery that yoga was to offer. Yes, I was finding out what my body rhythms and needs were, but I was also listening to my teacher as she told us about the ethics, principles, and guidelines. Not many teachers do this now, as yoga classes have become more of a popular exercise than a place to find out more about ourselves as we move, stretch, and meditate. But, there and then I was gifted with several teachers who introduced me to something deeper. My curiosity led me to become a yoga teacher. Becoming a yoga teacher led me to discovering the similarities between yoga and twelve-step recovery literature, which further led me to writing my first book, *Yoga and the Twelve-Step Path.*

If you are familiar with yoga, you will notice as you read *Yogic Tools for Recovery* that I have westernized the concepts and pointed them toward recovery. I did the same for myself when I utilized these ideas and ideals in my own process through the steps. I used some of these ideas working the steps with my sponsor, Bonnie R. (now deceased), and have used them in workshops and classes. I hadn't realized how much I had stuffed in my heart, in my muscles, and in my body until it started coming out. The physical yoga began to release "the issues in my tissues," and this new vocabulary let me work through it.

In my experience, I have found that the initial working of the steps is best done by the book, that is, using both the texts *Alcoholics Anonymous* and the *Twelve Steps and Twelve Traditions.* I believe this for a couple of reasons. One is that the majority of people in any twelve-step program are familiar with that process. Sponsors are well-versed in going through the steps in this fashion, and we develop a common language and a set of references to share with one another. I felt like I really belonged to my twelve-step group when I had completed the steps in the formal fashion. I then could speak at meetings with some authenticity. I learned what the multicolumn approach meant and understood what others were saying, allowing me to speak in the same terms. Having that shared experience made me part of the group.

Each of the steps has its own challenges to someone new in recovery. I was a recovery rebel, and I had objections for every step along the way. We who have held onto our lives and wits with stubborn tenacity might not understand how our lives were unmanageable. We might have seen that we were powerless over our addictive substance or behavior, but otherwise we held it all together. We might balk at the idea that we needed to be returned to sanity or that someone outside ourselves could care for us. The "higher-power thing" can be a huge stumbling block. Making a decision to turn our lives over to this entity we cannot understand or believe exists can be another hurdle in the process of recovery. When it comes to the working steps, in particular Steps Four through Nine, there are a lot of challenges that need to be faced. Looking at ourselves, asking for someone to witness our internal review, and acknowledging our hurts, harms, and destructive ways of living are all difficult. The dedication needed to make the list of people whom we have harmed and to winnow the list down to those whom we can and need to address is a process that requires the support of another person to help us find the meaningful *and* moderate path. The "maintenance steps"—Steps Ten, Eleven, and Twelve—also benefit from being done with the twelve-step program model and understanding. Down the road, it makes us better sponsors when we do.

Another reason I recommend the prescribed twelve-step recovery model is that as a newcomer, as someone who had pickled her brain out of any sense whatsoever, I needed to keep it simple. I had to avoid freestyling, doing it my own way. It was hard for me to understand and retain simple ideas. I needed the program to be explained in a clear and simple manner. I do that for my sponsees as well—we use the traditional language and a format that allows them to talk to others in the rooms with a common language and experience.

A few years into the program, when you are doing the steps for an additional time, you may be interested in looking at your life in a different way. Using the philosophy and guidance of yoga when working through the steps is for those wanting to look at that same work using a different lens.

My first time working the steps allowed me to get out the big chunks, the obvious and main issues facing me at that point. It is said that we aren't given anything we can't handle, and that was true for me. I was still fragile. I was insensate, meaning I was dull and addled in my mind. Not only were my emotions not ready to face the depth and subtlety of the "nature of my wrongs," but also I was incapable of seeing the more subtle aspects of these frailties.

It was later in recovery, once I had hit this new emotional bottom and when I was a little more mature, that I was ready to look deeper. I had to get over my mourning period. And, yes, in recovery we often go through the cycles of grief as we let go of our good-time self and become familiar with our new self in recovery. I needed to let good-time Kyczy go.

I was ready to embrace a new perspective on the woman I was becoming; I was able to see, more and more, how the defenses of the past were no longer working. I was ready to see that, even in recovery, I had wreckage to clean up, and I was ready to dig once again.

The philosophy and practice of yoga extend far beyond the mat practice, the poses, all that we associate with the word *yoga*. There are eight limbs of yoga as well as descriptions of our being, the challenges or sufferings and how they come to be, qualities of change and balance, and specific fields of energy within the body. All these concepts and ideas can be unpacked and described in relation to the process of addiction and recovery. An understanding of these concepts can enhance our view of the steps and provide another layer of unpeeling.

In the first two limbs of yoga, we begin with restraints and observances—the *yamas* and *niyamas,* respectively—that suggest a way to manage relationships with our self and with others. The five restraints could be considered the "traditions" of yoga: non-harming, non-lying, non-stealing, non-attachment, and non-excess or non-greed. Next, there are the observances, those qualities we follow to investigate and heal our insides, or the "steps" of yoga: cleanliness (of thought, speech, action, and health), contentment, discipline, study of one's self, and surrender.

The practice of the poses, or *asana,* when thoughtfully done, can teach us about the mind and allow us to develop and deepen our relationship with our body. From a deeper relationship with our physical being, we can begin to release trapped emotions and uncover hidden feelings.

Breath practices and control, or *pranayama,* can contribute a sense of mastery of our moods and energies and also provide a sense of peace. Carefully chosen and done under the tutelage of a trained instructor, this tool can be a powerful minister of change.

Withdrawal of the senses, letting go of that which has nothing to do with you, is one of the challenges in recovery. In yoga, we use this skill, also known as *pratyahara,* to notice and let go of the external world—sight, sound, smell, taste, touch—and continue the process in letting go of the scampering mind, the ultimate withdrawal of the senses.

Concentration—practicing the ability to focus—can be a huge challenge for people new to recovery. Regardless of where our paths have led us, "no matter how far down the scale we have gone," the ability to stay in the moment and to absorb the moment has been disturbed. It takes practice to return to or develop this skill, known as *dharana.*

Meditation, the suggestion of the Eleventh Step and the ultimate brain changer, is the seventh of the eight limbs of yoga. This is the culmination of all the restraints, observances, and practices. We have opened the possibility of treating others and ourselves with dignity and respect; we have learned to move and breathe and focus. It is now time to be still and listen.

The last limb of the eight limbs is *samadhi.* This is bliss and union with your higher power. It may manifest as being at one with all and being content with how things are in any given moment. It is the condition of having all illusions drop away and seeing the truth in all beings and all situations. It may be, for the blink of an eye, like our spiritual awakening—the event that opened our eyes to the truth, a truth that moved us beyond denial.

At some point before meditation or within meditation, the sufferings, or *kleshas,* emerge. These may appear as incorrect comprehension, ego, craving, avoidance, or fear. Facing these sufferings and moving through them can enlighten and awaken us to our new way a living; we may find we are truly "rocketed into a fourth dimension of existence."

Addiction is a holistic disease with three components: physical, mental, and spiritual. Yoga refines these three levels into five bodies, or *koshas:* energy, physical, emotional/mental, wisdom, and spiritual. The steps of recovery can be examined through the lens of impacts on each of these levels.

There are three subtle qualities of nature: sedentary, or stuck; movable, or active; and harmonious and balanced. In Sanskrit, these are called the *gunas*. Using this lens to evaluate a continuum of actions, feelings, and thoughts can inform and deepen one's experience with certain steps. They can provide a tool to evaluate emotional sobriety.

The seven main centers of spiritual power, the *chakras*, provide further information on where and how we hold onto and are affected by our disease. They can also provide a method to discern where work is yet to be done. Each chakra will express itself in a unique way when it is blocked or out of balance. Understanding the well-being of these centers can help us dig into the past with greater discernment and to process the issues of the present with more ease.

Yogic Tools for Recovery will explain and illustrate each of these concepts, and each of the twelve steps of recovery will be explored using the applicable precepts. This is an investigation and an additional tool that can augment the traditional way we work the steps. Grab a notebook, find a pen, give yourself some time, and travel with me. Enjoy the journey.

"Maybe you are searching among the branches
for what only appears in the roots."

RUMI

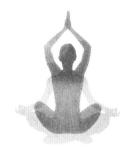

Acknowledgments

Every book is a big deal and takes proactive group support to bring it to publication; this one is no different. From tentative pieces that I tried out on friends in recovery to general sections that were presented to fellow authors, I was given encouragement to complete this work. I could not have done it alone.

I thank all of you who were able to read portions and provide feedback. This goes particularly to Anne Heffron, who throws up when she writes and made my process seem mild. Her laughter and incisive comments encouraged me to go ahead and speak from my heart when I write. Thank you to Wilson Ng, who urged me to be forthright, and to Shannon Stillman, whose affirmations I am grateful for. Every word helped.

I get a lot of support from my sister, Meridith Berk. She shares her work with me and comments on the bits and pieces I send to her. It is so wonderful to have a friend in my sister and to share the struggles of this often-solitary enterprise—writing—with her.

Thank you also to my recovery retinue who were unsuspecting guinea pigs while I unpacked the concepts used in this book—the development of the material. The Yoga Recovery meeting on ITR (In The Rooms) has helped me parse the subjects and guided me toward expressing myself clearly. My Friday night Y12SR (Yoga of 12 Step Recovery) group has added their experiences to expand and personalize the understanding of the yoga philosophy as it applies to all manner of recovery.

Thank you to the agencies that have invited me in to train personnel or lead classes for your clients. I have been able to expand my work from treatment centers to jails, to private for-profit agencies, and to private clients as the benefits of combining yoga and recovery are better understood. This experience has taught me that it really works! Yoga and recovery together can give you more and stronger strategies to avoid relapse. Together, we have come a long way in the last six years.

Experiences at my annual retreats have contributed to how the philosophies of yoga are intertwined step by step with recovery. I am thankful to all the attendees at the Santosha Retreats at the Land of Medicine Buddha. Your love and willingness to work through these ideas in that lovely group setting helped bring this book alive.

As important as a writer is to a book is the editor. Janet Ottenweller has been enthusiastic and supportive. Her organizational skills and ability to look at the work with perspective and care have transformed a relatively free-form, meandering work into a solid book. I am grateful to her in many ways; her being steadfast and affirming has helped this book take form.

I am grateful to the rhythm of my life; I have ample opportunity to write. I am grateful for the grace I have in my husband's support; I can write, erase, and write again, over and over, often neglecting him and his companionship. He is understanding as I pace around and gripe about the process. He just hangs in there, a voice of calm in the tempest of my mind.

Finally, I am grateful to all the yoga teachers who are expanding this practice across the states and around the world. I see more and more of you leading classes at conferences and retreats as well as studios and treatment centers. More and more people are able to experience the magic of coming home to one's true self with yoga.

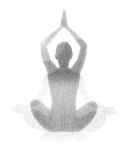

Introduction

YOGA TERMS AND PRINCIPLES

Yoga has a way of breaking down simple ideas, making them complex, and then making them simple again, which sounds a lot like recovery—the simple is not easy. Similar to recovery, yoga uses common words in new ways and expresses ideas in what might be thought of as jargon.

In recovery, we learn new ways to understand *surrender,* or letting go of the grip of our addiction. *Chips* are tokens for milestones, and are not made for dipping; *inventory* refers to characteristics and qualities, not items. We have specific ways in which we use phrases like *picking up* and *backsliding.* To the outsider, or without context, this terminology may be confusing or meaningless; however, these words and phrases—and countless others—are meaningful and fundamental to us in the way we communicate with others regarding the successes and perils of recovery.

So, too, yoga has words that are used in specific ways to convey deep meaning and ideas fundamental to the practice. We use words such as *energy, illusions,* and *self* in ways similar to and different from common usage. Concepts are combined to both integrate and differentiate groups of ideas.

In this book, I will relate the Sanskrit word and the more commonly used word from one of the many English translations. I will use English whenever possible for ease of understanding. The ideas are hard enough, the thoughts complex enough, so another layer of difficulty is not useful. My desire is to be clear and allow the intricacies of the concepts to unfold naturally. There are times when the English translation would be too long or lugubrious, so I will use the Sanskrit word instead. *Chakra* and *guna* are examples of these.

Patanjali is the name of the ancient sage who first transcribed the practice of yoga into written form. It had previously been a verbal tradition passed down from guru, or teacher, to student. There have been numerous translations over the years, not only into the various Indian dialects but also into most of the languages around the globe.

In addition to literal or transliteral translations, there are numerous commentaries and volumes of discourse on understandings of the brief aphorisms. I will be using the translations from various modern readings, while other *sutras,* or verses, have been adapted from the original Sanskrit word-for-word translations by me. The commentary will be my own as I reflect on the sutra and how it applies to recovery.

Kleshas

There are five kleshas, or sources of mental torment or sufferings: false understanding (*avidya*); ego (*asmita*); attachment/craving (*raga*); aversion (*dvesha*); and fear of change or death (*abhinivesha*). To illustrate them, one is often offered the image of a tree. The main suffering is depicted as the trunk, and the others are represented as the four limbs. As the original words are in Sanskrit, the English words used here are ones of many understandings.

Kleshas

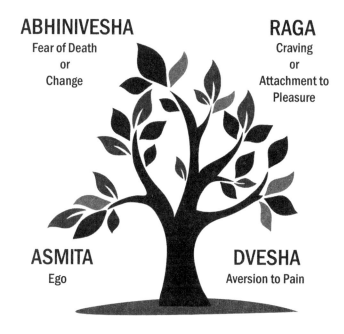

ABHINIVESHA
Fear of Death
or
Change

RAGA
Craving
or
Attachment to
Pleasure

ASMITA
Ego

DVESHA
Aversion to Pain

AVIDYA
False Understanding

False Understanding

The trunk of the tree, false understanding or avidya, is the base. According to Sutra 2.4, "Spiritual ignorance (avidya) is the cause of the kleshas whether they are dormant, weak, interrupted, or sustained." Denial, the state of being before we take the First Step, is a perfect example of this misery. We see the untrue as true, the transitory as permanent, and we mistake pain for pleasure. It is a lack of awareness, not a permanent blindness. We often say, "When we know better, we do better." This phrase exemplifies our ability to change. We talk about a spiritual experience that allows us to see things clearly; the veil or scales fall from our eyes, the denial fades, and we come to. Then, we have a new sector of life, relationships, and challenges, and we again have faulty vision and suffer from a false understanding.

We don't always need to wait for a spiritual experience or a tragic event to wake us up. As I have moved through recovery, I have found that there are signs, events, or visceral responses to activities that announce an opportunity to become aware. Yoga practice and meditation can often lead me to change, amend, and renew my understanding of people, places, and things. I use the lens of false understanding to evaluate what I am experiencing, and then I can make a choice. This is a human condition, and I remind myself it is not a one-and-done experience. I remain open to the possibility that I don't understand a situation fully, and that "more will be revealed."

Ego

The first limb we come to on the tree is asmita—ego, or false sense of self. Sutra 2.6, which discusses this limb, can be translated as "Egoism is the identification of the Seer (Parusha) with the sense organs," meaning we identify ourselves with how we appear or how we feel. We incorrectly ignore the true self, the eternal self, that lies within us. In active addiction and even in early recovery, we can be so identified with our actions and behaviors as someone compelled to use or act in injurious ways that we forget our true self. We may identify with the persona that seeks to protect our addict self to the neglect of our internal values. What is the true "me"? It is a concept that is often discussed at meetings and struggled through with sponsors.

You may have seen the sign on twelve-step meeting room walls that reads, "Think, Think, Think." In early recovery we have been told that it doesn't apply to us, as our "thinkers are broken." I was confused. I read the sign and heard people say, "My best thinking got me here." So should I think or not? "Think things through" might have been a better sign for me.

This wisdom from recovery can be emphasized by the yoga sutras that suggest that we not confuse what we think with who we are—our mental impressions and our true self. I learned to perceive things in a new way in recovery, reversing the false impressions I was under when I drank and used. While intoxicated, I thought I was an expert in all things, the wittiest and most amiable of all, super sexy and desirable. These were cover-ups and exaggeration, not, in any way, how I truly felt. To refer again to Sutra 2.6, I was identifying as my *false* self—that part of me that I thought about, or that part of me I wished to represent to others. I had forgotten my true self.

The *Twelve Steps and Twelve Traditions* by Alcoholics Anonymous includes the following quote about our misuse of ego: "The problem is to help them discover a chink in the walls their ego has built, through which the light of reason can shine." The perception of ego is compared to a wall, and we are looking for a small crack or opening through which the light of reason and, one could say, true spirit can shine.

I am in the grip of the false ego when I am in active addiction. I am not making choices and decisions from my internal *atman,* or true self. I am operating under the illusion of my using self, the one who changes standards, who changes values, preferences, and dreams to support the gnawing need of *more.* I don't save money for rent; I don't act in a respectful way to others or myself; I don't care. I don't care at all about anything but getting my next whatever—pair of shoes, hand of cards, sexual conquest, drink, fix, or pill. I am not me; I am an active addict.

In recovery, I can also fall into a false sense of self. This happens when I identify so strongly with a role, a job, a clothing size, an age, or something else to such a degree that I lose sight of my being. When I restrict myself to a certain aspect of being, in body, mind, or spirit, I lose sense of my greater connection to my higher power. Whether that self-concept is too big *or* too little, it is a false sense of self. The steps help me evaluate and investigate these illusions of ego.

Attachment/Craving

The next limb of the tree is raga, or attachment or craving. Sutra 2.7 states, "Attachment is that which rests upon pleasant experiences." Doesn't that sound like another way of describing addiction? I used initially to make myself happy; later, I used to prevent myself from feeling at all. This attachment in its extreme form is used to cover existential terror, the fear and feeling that what one perceives is real and overwhelming, painful, or dangerous. It is the false thinking we crave that protects us from our own thoughts and feelings, and we think it will protect us from others. In the intense throes of addiction, nothing else matters. This is the hell we sink into before we attempt to find recovery. The phrase *no matter how far down the scale we have gone* describes the condition perfectly. We do not have to go to hospitals, jails, or institutions to have descended into hell. It is a personal state of misery, shame, and helplessness.

Even in recovery, we can find attachments to things such as a job, a person, or another slice of cake. We may counteract the feelings of not being enough by trying to have more: more money, a bigger or better house, a faster car, a luxury vacation, an antique collection, or a greater status of any kind. We may be looking for external forces or factors to protect our fragile inner self. These protections, too, are illusions that we discover either when we achieve them or when we don't, or when we have them or when we lose them. Attachments will fail us; when we put our power and identity in "people, places, and things," we forget our real self.

Aversion

Situations that once caused us pain may be avoided in the future. We can stop trying new things if we are initially ignored or belittled by our efforts. I may decide not to get into a romantic relationship with another person due to a betrayal. The avoidance of situations that follow the experience of pain is called dvesha, or aversion, the third limb of the tree. Sutra 2.8 explains, "Aversion is that which rests upon sorrowful experiences." The experience can be directly felt as an actual one, or it can be the result of a story told so often that you think it is the truth. It could be as simple as being told you don't look good in a certain color, and you take that as the truth for years. It is an antipathy toward something long after the event or ordeal. Even after circumstances have changed, and long after the occurrence, a "bad taste in your mouth" lingers from the memory.

In a simple case, it might indeed be a taste: a vegetable, a flavor, even an entire type of cuisine. You may never want to eat fish, brussels sprouts, or Brie cheese. It could be a type of entertainment, such as water slides or roller coasters. It may be reading for leisure or exercising for fun. Something happened one time, and it caused a negative reaction that you were unable to rebound from. You had to stay at the table or be shamed by others about not eating all your food. You may have had a fear of high places and been forced to try an amusement park ride, regardless of your feelings, never to try one again. You could have found reading difficult, and the pleasure was punished out of you. We avoid pain.

Feelings of discomfort, the consequences of having others' disapproval, and the fear of physical harm can conspire in you to cause an aversion so great that you will do anything to avoid them. When actions and attitudes won't cover the pain, we believe engaging in one's addiction surely will; however, it is not a conscious choice. A person may say, "I hate the way I am feeling, so I will drink," but what he or she means is that drinking allowed those feelings to go away, so he or she will do it again.

As we say in the rooms of recovery, it is more than abstinence. We have work to do, deep down, so we can heal. We start by "putting the plug in the jug" of whatever form of substance or behavior our addiction takes. If we don't do that, we won't get anywhere in recovery. And, we won't get anywhere with the steps.

Life continues to offer challenges where we can investigate aversion in the forms of dissatisfaction, reluctance, and unwillingness.

As we learn to live one day at a time, our trials can be turned into miracles when we find the courage to face them.

Fear

The last and fourth limb on the tree of afflictions is abhinivesha, or the fear of death or change. Sutra 2.9 states, "Clinging to life, even the sages flow along with its own momentum." This insecurity and anxiety referred to in the sutra—sometimes translated as fear and other times specifically as fear of death—are pervasive throughout humanity. We addicts seem to have a withering dose of it. Whether it is fear of death or of a more minor change, our first reaction is dread, mistrust, and dis-ease. The Big Book describes this reaction to fear perfectly with the phrase *restless, irritable, and discontent*.

In a life circumstance of uncertainty, I used to retreat into fear. It often was expressed as anger and resistance. Working through the steps on many aspects of my recovery has given me perspective. I have practiced looking at the world with more faith, trust, peace, and joy. I am now able to use the information of feeling fear to direct me toward a deeper excavation of my perceptions and false understanding, which allows me to uncover the source, the seminal event that may underlie my current reaction.

Reducing Kleshas

The section of the yogic writings beginning with Sutra 2.2 provides hope: "The practice of Kriya Yoga reduces the afflictions (kleshas) and leads toward *samadhi*." As we practice, the way will become clear, as will our perceptions. Just as we use the Twelve Steps to clear our understanding, we can use the afflictions to understand ourselves in conjunction with the steps.

Sutras 2.10 and 2.11 inform us that "*pratiprasava* is overcoming the five afflictions in the subtle form by resolving them backward to their origin," and that "meditation will overcome the fluctuations of the consciousness caused by the afflictions." With the Eleventh Step, we advance to this suggested yogic state of reflection through prayer and meditation.

The program of recovery suggests we continue to "practice these principles in all our affairs." This is the idea that our practice is never quite complete. Once again, the ancient knowledge and understanding of yoga underline and underlie the wisdom of twelve-step fellowships.

Koshas

One of the translations of the word *yoga* is "union of body, mind, and spirit." This lines up perfectly with the Alcoholics Anonymous statements that we have "a physical allergy, a mental obsession, and a spiritual malady." Yoga and twelve-step recovery are indeed a perfect match. On further examination, however, yoga actually goes a little deeper, refining the body and mind layers into two pieces each.

The koshas, or layers of our being, begin with the physical layer, the only kosha visible to the eye (*annamaya kosha*). We then move to the energy layer (*pranamaya kosha*). This layer is the energy that keeps the fluid and air moving, as well as what yogis refer to as the subtle energies of the body. The subtle energies drive the various rhythms of our being, such as respiration and other cycles of movement in the body.

The layers related to the mind are the mental/emotional layer (*manomaya kosha*) and the wisdom layer (*vijnanamaya kosha*). The former holds our emotions while the latter holds our character, or our witness self.

The final layer is the spirit or bliss layer (*anandamaya kosha*). We experience bliss, union, and community of wholeness in this fifth layer. When we are in sync with our higher power, we are experiencing this in the spiritual layer of our being.

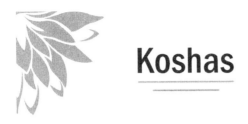

Koshas

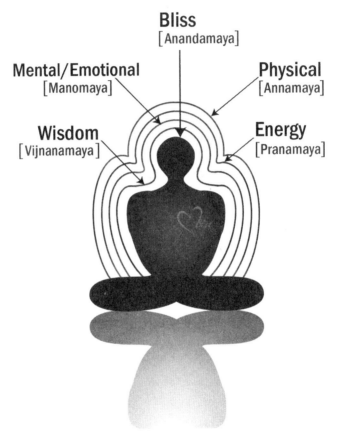

Bliss
[Anandamaya]

Mental/Emotional
[Manomaya]

Physical
[Annamaya]

Wisdom
[Vijnanamaya]

Energy
[Pranamaya]

Each of these layers communicates with the others. If one layer is stressed, it may impact another one. If you are tired (energy layer), you may also feel achy or vaguely ill (physical layer). When your feelings are hurt (emotional layer), you may feel tight and uncomfortable in your physical layer. And, you may feel disconnected from your spiritual layer when you are uncomfortable or in pain in any of the other four layers.

HALT and the Koshas

In recovery, we use the acronym HALT, which stands for Hungry, Angry, Lonely, or Tired. These four states are the origins of triggers that can make us vulnerable to relapse, and they can be correlated to the koshas.

The physical layer lets us know if we are hungry—the first part of HALT. It also records tension, relaxation, anger, and release from anger. Our ability to move, stretch, and run from and run to is facilitated by our physical layer. This layer also retains the fingerprints, or shadows, from our emotions. If we are unable to process the physical or emotional events that have happened to us, they become lodged as stuck energy. This energy will reside in the physical body—in our muscles, tendons, ligaments, and nervous system. The energy layer will be affected as well.

The energy layer records the "electricity" of events, or the charge that remains in us long after an event has passed. The nervous system knows no time—meaning memories are recorded as the present. If you hear a song, you can sometimes feel as you felt the first time you heard it. Images, smells, and feelings can all come rushing back. This can happen in a positive as well as a negative way. This layer also manifests in sensations such as being tired—the T of HALT. When we are tired, we may bump into things, our breath may not be full, or our temper and the way we express it may become harsh or snappy. Depletion or being out of balance in this layer can have far-reaching effects on other layers.

The emotional layer is the part that can be seen as connecting the physical and energy layers with the nervous system. This is how the body-mind association is made—our physical sensations become our emotional feelings. This layer is like a control panel or a fuse box bringing the physical pulses into the brain. We sense; we process; we record. If we sense with false glasses, we record incorrect information. Sometimes, the processor doesn't discern correct from incorrect thinking, or we have other afflictions that cause an override of wiser thought. One day, being alone is wonderful: we can read, choose our meals, and come and go as we please. Another day, being alone may feel lonely and possibly unloved. And on yet another day, we may sink into a feeling of separation and isolation. Another situation could arise when we are left with a feeling of annoyance that is small and manageable. Another day, these same feelings may be overwhelming, and we may burst into anger. These situations and responses are examples of the A and L of HALT reflected in the layers of being.

The wisdom kosha is the layer that reflects on what is going on. This part notices that it is knowing, sees what it is viewing. This layer is where reasoning happens. When we are tired, this layer tells us to rest, and when we are hungry, it tells us to eat. When we are troubled, it can advise us to connect with our spirit layer and higher power. The wisdom layer is also there to compare and discern, considering information that is coming from the world around us. These considerations help us make choices.

The bliss, or spirit, layer is the part of ourselves that we bring to prayer and meditation, and it is also impacted by the other layers of being. When we think of Hungry, Angry, Lonely, and Tired as conditions, they can sever a strong relationship with the spirit self. In yoga, as in our recovery fellowship, we look to the bliss layer to detach from difficulties, identify troubles, and find resources to bring us back to balance—all five bodies with the spirit.

When we find balance, we are able to fully connect with bliss. One of the ways we can involve the heart in this healing process is to use the chakras.

Chakras

There are seven main energy centers in the body called chakras. There is no simple English word for *chakra,* and "energy center in the body" is too long to repeat, so I will use the Sanskrit word. While we think of the chakras as being in certain loci along the spine, the influence of the energy of each roams around the body in specific areas. Each chakra has a prevalent color, tone, or sound and specific ways it manifests when stuck or overactive.

Chakras

1
2
3
4
5
6
7

CHAKRA NAME	IN BALANCE	OUT OF BALANCE	ASSOCIATED WITH THIS PART OF THE BODY	NATURAL HEALING
CROWN	SPIRITUALITY / HARMONY / CONNECTION	INDECISIVE, LACK CREATIVITY AND JOY	METABOLISM, SPINE / NECK/ HEAD, "DNA"	MEDITATION, STAR GAZING, WATCHING CLOUDS
THIRD EYE	AWARENESS	UNDISCIPLINED, MEEK, FEARFUL OF SUCCESS	CENTRAL NERVOUS SYSTEM, ENDOCRINE SYSTEM	DREAMING, VISION BOARDS, FOCUSED IMAGININGS
THROAT	COMMUNICATION	INCONSISTENT, UNABLE TO EXPRESS THOUGHTS / TRUTH, UNRELIABLE	THYROID, PARATHYROID, RESPIRATORY SYSTEM	SINGING, CHANTING, READING ALOUD, DISCUSSION WITH OTHERS
HEART	LOVE, HEALING, COMPASSION	INDECISIVE, SELF PITY, DOUBTFUL, FEARFUL	HEART, LUNGS, LYMPH	SELF CARE AND COMPASSION, CHALLENGING GROWTH
SOLAR PLEXUS	WISDOM, POWER, SELF CONFIDENCE	LACK OF PERSONAL ENERGY, LOW SELF ESTEEM, LACK OF CONFIDENCE	DIGESTION, STOMACH, LIVER,	SUNSHINE, HEALTHY ACTIVITIES, BEING IN NATURE
SACRAL	SEXUALITY, SENSUALITY	LACK OF INTIMACY, FEAR, SEXUAL GUILT, SHYNESS	SPLEEN, URINARY TRACT, ALSO KIDNEYS	CREATIVE EXPRESSION, ART, MUSIC, ETC.
ROOT	STABILITY, TRUST	SCATTERED THOUGHTS	LEGS, FEET, KIDNEYS, BLOOD	GROUNDING, SETTLING, SECURITY

Each chakra is related to a physical condition and system in the body. There are certain provisions and challenges manifested by each energy center. While there are many subtle chakras in the body, we will be focusing on only seven of the main "wheels," or spinning spheres of energy, and how each manifests in both overactivity and underactivity.

Knowing these conditions will be of great use when doing the Fourth, Sixth, and Seventh Steps of recovery. Additionally, each chakra influences both the emotional and physical layers of being, or koshas.

Root Chakra

The root chakra is of fundamental importance. This first chakra is located at the base of the spine and governs our sense of security, our basic survival needs, and our senses of safety and connection. Physical disturbances in this chakra can manifest in a variety of ways, including constipation, disordered eating, sciatica, knee pain, and arthritis. Signs of emotional imbalance can show up as hoarding or greed and lack of discipline or fearfulness, among other security-related feelings.

Sacral Chakra

The sacral, or second, chakra is located along the spine behind the low belly, just under the navel. It governs our abilities to be playful, creative, intimate, and committed, as well as our sexuality. When it is activated excessively, we may be overly emotional or have poor boundaries in relationships in terms of both intimacy and sexuality. When this chakra is underactivated, we may feel the opposite: rigid, without playfulness, fearful of betrayal, and even having a tendency toward addiction. Physically, imbalance shows up in our lower back, hip area, kidneys, and reproductive organs.

Solar Plexus Chakra

The solar plexus chakra is located about five inches above the sacral chakra, three or four finger widths above the navel. This is the seat of our will, our power center, and our sense of effectiveness in the world. When the solar plexus chakra is overactive, emotional imbalances occur, such as hubris, control issues, and a need to criticize others. When it is underactive, imbalances may appear as poor self-esteem, passivity, fearfulness, and having an overactive inner critic. The physical impacts of an out-of-balance third chakra can be digestive problems, fatigue, high blood pressure, or diabetes.

The stomach, pancreas, and other organs can be impacted as well. When operating in equilibrium, the solar plexus chakra allows us to feel balanced and have self-respect and self-compassion. We have appropriate boundaries and an adequate amount of confidence.

Heart Chakra

The fourth chakra, the heart chakra, is located, yes, behind your heart. When it is balanced, we have a secure sense of joy, love, compassion, gratitude, and forgiveness. When it is overactive, we may be codependent, feel jealousy, be clingy, and/or fear abandonment. It is another area where we may lose wise boundaries. If it is underactive, we may isolate, withdraw from others, or lack forgiveness or compassion. Some of the physical associations of this chakra are the lymph nodes, upper back, shoulders, arms, and wrists. The respiratory and lymphatic systems may be involved as well.

Throat Chakra

The throat chakra governs our communication, including our ability to express our truth. The physical connections include thyroid issues, throat health, ear health, and facial and upper-back issues. When in balance, the throat chakra allows us easy speech and expression, right communication, and the ability to speak honestly without harm. We also have the skill of listening. If this chakra is underactive, we may have poor speech rhythm, a sore throat as the result of swallowing our words, a fear of power or making choices, or lack of power in expressing self to the world. If the throat chakra is overactive, we have too loud a volume, use rapid speech, talk over others, or interrupt.

Third Eye Chakra

Between and just above the eyebrows is where the sixth chakra rests. The third eye chakra relates to our intuition, imagination, and focus. We can tell the difference between real and unreal, between truth and illusion. Some of the things this chakra governs are our vision, sinus, hearing, and hormone functions. An overactive third eye chakra can manifest as headaches, nightmares, difficulty concentrating, or daydreaming. With an underactive sixth chakra, one may have poor memory or an inability to see patterns, learn from others, or even look at ourselves.

Crown Chakra

The crown, or seventh, chakra is located on the top of the head when sitting upright. A balanced crown chakra allows us to live in the present moment, to feel connection to others and the universe. We may have a free-flowing sense of unity with our higher power. We have confidence and trust in our inner guidance system. This chakra governs our emotional well-being and our ability to learn. We are in harmony with our five senses.

A physical imbalance can include depression, an impaired ability to learn, and a heightened sensitivity to light, sight, sound, or touch—the environment in general. When the seventh chakra is overactive, we experience an emotional imbalance and may retreat into the mind, becoming overly intellectual, perhaps spiritually rigid or confused. We may experience "analysis paralysis," that state of staying in the brain rather than thinking wholeheartedly. The underactive seventh chakra may manifest in limited beliefs, skepticism, or even learning difficulties. We may carry unexamined prejudices and have difficulty with self-knowledge. And we may become depressed.

Recovery and Chakras

Evaluating ourselves through the Twelve Steps using the lens of the chakra system requires both an easy hand and a global view. As with the steps, where we work them in sequence, it is important to start with the first chakra—the root—and work up. Each one has its own importance and rests upon the one before it.

As we work the steps, I will offer ways to evaluate the chakras, where applicable, and their impact on the steps. They do not stay stable—either in or out of balance—but there are ways to note the impact of the chakras on our daily life.

Gunas

There are three qualities that underlie all of nature: sedentary, sluggish, dark, and slow-moving; movable, mutable, and active; and stable and harmonious. In Sanskrit these are known as the *tamas, rajas,* and *sattva;* the states are called *tamasic, rajasic,* and *sattvic.* These qualities are not good or bad; they exist. There is movement among the three; however, it is when we get stuck in tamas or rajas that we experience difficulties.

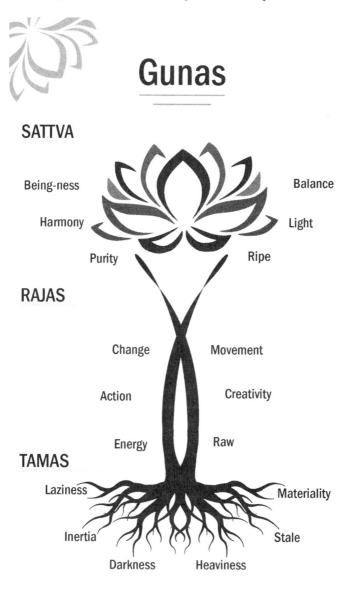

Gunas

SATTVA

Being-ness   Balance

Harmony   Light

Purity   Ripe

RAJAS

Change   Movement

Action   Creativity

Energy   Raw

TAMAS

Laziness   Materiality

Inertia   Stale

Darkness   Heaviness

We can view almost all of life through the lenses of these qualities: colors, behaviors, tastes, and sounds. All the senses reflect the influence of these conditions. Going back to the chakras, we can see tamasic or rajasic qualities in the out-of-balance conditions; excess and deficient qualities can be interpreted by the lack of harmony in the expression of emotions and physical wellness.

Tamas

Tamas can prevent us from seeing the needs of others and being oblivious, perhaps, to our own health and wellness needs. After a period of self-oriented overdoing—succumbing to our addiction— we may wake up in the morning in a tamasic state of loathing, pity, and illness. It can also be discerned as an unwillingness to change— at any point in recovery. There may be a heavy weight or pull of being toward old behavior and not wanting, or feeling unable, to change. Tamas is useful in order to get us to the point of being "sick and tired of being sick and tired."

Rajas

We need rajas to move us. There is no way to move from the deep-denial part of addiction to the harmony we feel from time to time in recovery without the energy of rajas. While rajas can be seen as restless action and activity, it is also the energy needed for change. In excess, this rajasic energy is unfocused movement, covering emotions and distractions from growth. It can also be seen as a catapult to move from here to there thoughtfully. It only becomes problematic when we stay in movement for the sake of motion, without action to move us to harmony.

Sattva

Imagine the steadfast nature and wisdom of Yoda from Star Wars. This is sattva. Virtue, goodness, and intelligence, together with creating harmony, are aspects of this quality. It is a "moving toward" without judgment or criticism, which is most helpful in acquiring this state of being; however, it doesn't last. It is, again, practice, not perfection. Sattva is happiness and contentment of an enduring nature. Returning time and time again to sattva is part of the "mini-miracles" of recovery.

Yamas and Niyamas

The yamas and the niyamas are the practices that precede the postures, breath control, meditation, and the ultimate union with our higher power. These principles are indispensable when working the steps as well as in living a yogic life. These ten concepts begin in our value system and are practiced on several levels: thought, word, and action. Using the following quote from Gandhi as a paradigm, one can see the importance of these ideals.

Your beliefs become your thoughts,

Your thoughts become your words,

Your words become your actions,

Your actions become your habits,

Your habits become your values,

Your values become your destiny.

The yamas, or restraints, are classified as non-harming, non-lying, non-stealing, non-excess, and non-attachment (*ahimsa, satya, asteya, brahmacharya,* and *aparigraha*). The niyamas, or observances, are known as cleanliness, contentment, self-study, discipline, and surrender (*saucha, santosha, svadhyaya, tapas,* and *ishvara pranidhana*). These values mirror many that we already find in recovery. Focusing step work in relation to yamas and niyamas can help identify areas that are troublesome or areas in which we have made improvements already. Each of these values is also fairly complex, referring not only to people, places, and things but also ideas, time, and energy.

These ethics or scruples can be taken together or examined as we interact with another person. For example, one can harm both oneself and another by stealing his or her wallet, affection, attention, or credit for his or her work. One can also steal someone's time or care by asking for help and then misusing it. Harm and stealing have interacted here. Not keeping your side of the street clean in your relationships and interchanges can also result in harm, hurt feelings, unresolved arguments, or apologies missed. There is no restraint being practiced when you find yourself walking off with the last word, to the detriment of the other person.

Each one of the yamas and niyamas will be developed in detail as we move through the steps in the coming chapters. Having the basic ideas with the basic levels of practice—thought, word, and action—will provide much help when working the steps and unraveling our behavior. Without these values, our lifelong yoga practice has neither balance nor legs, and recovery will topple as well.

Karma

Our actions and the intentions of our actions have outcomes. These outcomes, whether they occur right away or in the future, are known as *karma*. Karma results from both positive and negative deeds and behaviors, whether done purposely or not, and no matter the motivation, plan, or design. Encompassed within the idea of consequence is that we let go of, or have no control over, the outcome. In recovery, we let go. We do the footwork of action and let our higher power take it from there.

Seva

Service, or *seva,* is a very important part of our recovery path, which can be enfolded into our amends. It can contribute to developing self-esteem and help us become aware of our usefulness in the world. From greeter to secretary, from someone who sweeps the studio floor to someone who washes the mats, we are in service in our yoga and recovery communities—and, eventually, in communities beyond.

Kula

My addiction wants me alone; it wants me fearful and hopeless. My addiction hides in unlikely places and takes different forms. My drinking could masquerade as sex; it could look like a job I couldn't leave or a break I couldn't take. My addiction keeps me from being with my community, or *kula,* in healthy communion with life around me.

My antidote to the isolation in which my addiction wants me to dwell is my yoga practice and my recovery. It is to find healthy company and associate with people who are "doing the deal," "walking the walk," and, as my friend Shashi says, "staying in the middle of the herd." I can still feel lonely or afraid, or have bouts of hopelessness and insecurity, but when I practice my discipline (tapas), I reconnect with others, reach outside myself, and become part of something again. Together, we will evaluate the power of community as we do the steps.

Samskara

Our memories and the thought patterns and habits they create invade our field of awareness in the present. You may or may not be conscious of the memories for them to still have an impact. When you become aware of them, you can choose how to respond or react to them. Our memories and reactions conspire together to make habits in the mind, or *samskara*. These habits can be experienced on all levels of our being: physical; energy; emotional; wisdom; and, possibly, spiritual. An example of the sensory habit can be simple, such as the smell of an orange when you peel the fruit, causing your mouth to salivate in anticipation. If you are in the habit of ringing a chime at the beginning of meditation, just hearing the bell can bring a sense of calm. On the other end of the spectrum, if you have lived in a war-torn area and you hear a car door slam, you may jump with adrenaline coursing through your body. A loud, abrupt sound can trigger feelings from the past.

On a more complex level, seeing a bar scene in a movie may romance the idea of drinking and bring to mind a subtle craving and emotions. Some scenes or episodes of shows may be too overwhelming and incite a craving too strong, so that the show itself must be shunned in order to avoid increasing the rut, the habit of the mind, from continuing down that path to dis-ease.

The habits of the mind, like any habit, can become an "easier, softer way" when not examined. The patterns of codependency—the people pleasing, the fear of authority, the silencing of your own wishes and dreams, to name a few—can be reflexive actions. Even though these actions hurt us, we still do them.

Additionally, when we become lazy and avoid self-reflection, we may fall into thought patterns from the past that result in unhealthy actions. Relapse may result. Luckily, acknowledging and healing these habits of the mind is what the steps of recovery were designed to address.

Asana

The physical postures of yoga are referred to as asana. The translation is actually "seat" but is broadly referred to as "the poses." There are many lineages of yoga and modifications for all the poses, yet they all fall under the category of asana.

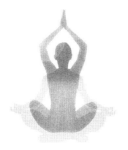

Chapter One

SETTING THE STAGE

— STEP ONE —

We admitted that we were powerless over our addiction,
that our lives had become unmanageable.

Addiction is best described by the opening of Charles Dickens's *A Tale of Two Cities:* "It was the best of times; it was the worst of times." An activity that once had been the source of enjoyment, respite, distraction, attraction, fun, and freedom had now become the essence of despair, pain, guilt, illness, and shame. Whatever the craving—gambling, spending, food, sex, relationships, drugs, or booze—the pain now eclipsed the pleasure to an insurmountable degree.

These painful feelings are the source of the knee-buckling desperation that comes before the First Step. In the rooms of recovery, we call this "the step before the steps," that moment of incomprehensible demoralization that gives you the gift of desperation to be willing to give it up—whatever *it* is. The desire to stop is the only requirement for membership in any recovery program.

At this point, you become ready to do whatever it takes and begin the First Step of recovery. You want to feel better, think more clearly, and get the monkey off your back; however, the path to long-term recovery may not be smooth. When the reality of abstinence sets in, when the mind and body feel better, resistance to sobriety and abstinence may descend from "whatever it takes" to becoming belligerent and making deals with recovery, possibly thinking that active addiction wasn't that bad. A few weeks into feeling better, I was ready to barter.

For Karen, a friend in recovery, the resistance arose first from the idea that she could never use or drink again. Next, she fought the concept that she would need to go to meetings and share with others. Reminded that it is a "we" program, she felt uneasy with the thought that she was now part of a group. Her strength had always been in doing things herself. With little family support, even from a young age, she found self-sufficiency her strongest character trait—an attribute she cherished. When it was appropriate to assert her independence, her approach had been based on the "I do!" statement of a toddler, which later in life became a liability.

Due to issues with control that were based on incidents and events in her youth, Karen was doubtful about putting her trust in others, even as a newly sober person. The "What do you mean *we*? I have been doing *fine* on my own" attitude could isolate her. Gaining trust and remaining teachable would be the touchstones of her recovery.

Like Karen, I waffled between surrender and control. When I floundered, wise people in recovery didn't try to talk me out of my feelings. They helped me examine the outcome of my life-management techniques. My health was a wreck, my family life was coming apart, I was financially impoverished, and I didn't have a safe place for my children and me to live. This was the control I was unwilling to give up. It took some time, but I settled down and settled in.

Later my feelings would flip, and I would be happy about being part of a group. I was profoundly lonely and experienced a dull ache of constant separation from people; I had no sense of place or belonging.

There were moments when that deep sense of separation would lift, and the idea of being part of a community—part of a fellowship—was appealing. I would toggle between the two feelings, thinking I could do this on my own and having the relief of being part of something.

Additional arrogance would soon descend as I became offended by the word *powerless*. For goodness' sake! I could barely dress myself; I looked like a crone. I was under thirty and disheveled, bloated, rheumy eyed, mentally unstable, and unhealthy in all ways. This was not the powerful woman I imagined in my mind, the haughty and self-righteous being who thought she was in control.

As a woman coming of age in the late 1960s and early 1970s, fighting for the right to make decisions by and for myself, I embraced the rallying cry of the time. It was the age of women's rights, racial rights, and power to the people, and having power—in whatever shape or form I imagined it—was part of my struggle to become a person. The word *power* was loaded in a way I don't think the founders of AA had imagined; it triggered ideas of selfhood, which I took out of context. Eventually, I calmed down and realized that I was not relinquishing *all* power, just power over my substances.

Additionally, I found fault with the word *unmanageable*. I managed my drinking and using. I just barely managed to buy booze and score dope, which was the maximum of my capacity to manage. I also managed to make a mess of my life and the lives of my children and other people whom I loved and cared about. I had to let go of the idea that I had been managing my life adequately.

The other huge part of manageability that I lacked was the ability to handle my internal world. I didn't know the difference between an impulse and a well-thought-out plan that included an awareness of consequences. I didn't know how to identify and contend with my emotions, good or bad. Love for another was an obsession, fear was debilitating, worry became apprehension, and anticipation became misery. There was no dimmer switch on my feelings: I was hysterically happy, deep in fear, or paralyzed with anxiety. If the outer world was bad, the inner world was devastating.

I kept defending my life with stories about what I *could* manage without looking at those parts I couldn't. It was clear I couldn't manage my emotions, my reactions, and my craving. Yet, I resisted. I don't know why I held on so tightly to the idea that I could manage my life; it could have been that I needed to retain a thread of self-esteem in order to feel worthy of recovery. I don't know. But as many newcomers do, I had to perseverate over how wrong the words of the First Step were until I could accept them as being right. Unfortunately, this unwillingness continues to pop up, even now in later recovery. I struggle with the difference between what I can and cannot do for and by myself.

It took me years to really *listen* to Step One: it states that I am powerless over my substances, not that I am without power. I had the power to change, the power to let go, and the power to believe. Now, I have all sorts of power. I lack power only over my addictive substances and behaviors. The rest of the world is my oyster—a yummy one, in fact.

Eventually, I was able to take this step in earnest and at all levels. I became part of a group, and I let go of the idea that I could control, much less enjoy, using or drinking, because the seams of my life had frayed. I was ready to change. I used the guidance of my fellowship's primary texts to do this.

Later in recovery, I would do the steps, all of them, again—several times. I moved multiple times to accommodate jobs and needed to establish relationships with new sponsors. Reworking the steps was a way to do this. One's point of view and depth of investigation change over time. This was true for me, too. I was able to dig a little deeper and uncover subtle details, motivations, and consequences more thoroughly than when I first worked the steps.

In recent years, as I have become more steeped in yoga in all its forms, I have looked at the steps with my yogic tools. I have found that steps can be approached with the paradigm of yogic philosophy. I reapplied myself to working all the steps, starting, of course, with Step One.

Using many of the yamas and the kleshas and evaluating the impact on the koshas and the chakras, I worked the First Step. The gunas have their place as well as we move from the darkest states to the practice of living a life in harmony. Referring to the definitions and explanations in the introduction may assist in this discussion.

Yamas and Step One

The yamas, or restraints, that are addressed during the First Step are non-harming, non-excess, and non-attachment.

Non-harming

The step before the steps, the readiness to embark on a new way of life, came at that point when the reality that I was harming myself became undeniable. I was in all manner of pain: physical, mental, emotional, financial, and spiritual. I could no longer deny that the harm I was doing to myself was also hurting others. The only way to stop this harm was to stop using and drinking.

In later recovery, I have faced other obsessions and delusions. In my early years, I had been quite codependent in all my relationships, including those with my children, my parents, my boyfriend, and my boss. When I reworked the steps with non-harming in mind, I realized I was taking away others' dignity in giving them unsolicited solutions to their problems, denying them the privilege of working their own way through issues. By not having boundaries, I was hurting myself as well as others, allowing them to ask more of me than was reasonable and asking myself to give more than was healthy. I would then fall into anger or rage because this overaccommodation was not returned. I took on a martyr's role in thinking the world owed me something because I couldn't say no.

Non-excess

I was violating the ethic of non-excess on a daily basis in my drinking and using habits. I had, as many people say in recovery, the "disease of more." Starting from the time when using and drinking had been a form of recreation until it became a form of self-preservation, I had always been attracted to more.

In redoing the steps, I found that there were many areas where "more" had seemed better than "some": approval, activity, and busyness, to name a few. I found that working the First Step on excesses let me see how these issues were running my life, and not in a healthy or reasonable way.

Non-attachment

I was attached to old ideas, or concepts, of what was good and bad. I was committed to my drinking and using buddies and, in a confused way, to my old way of living. I was attached to my illusions of control, wrong thinking, and dis-eased perceptions of life. I wanted things to change, but I also wanted them to remain the same.

There are times when I still hold on. I hold onto winning an argument, having the last word, and being in the front of the class or in the back of the line. These times are not as frequent or as intense now. I pause and reflect, but I realize something deep down still needs work. When I have concepts of myself that I hold onto that are not salutary, or when I hold onto the idea that the only way something will get done is for it to be done by me, these are also occasions of backsliding that remind me that I am not "cured." This is attachment of the most conceited type—as if only I could manage or perform certain jobs. This yama of non-attachment helps me find humility.

Kleshas and Step One

The sufferings, or afflictions, in my life were many and voluminous; the shame, the guilt, the fear, the insecurity, the danger, and the mayhem were overwhelming. But, somehow, I had become accustomed to them, so I was fearful of change. This was a conflict that consumed much of what little energy I had in moving toward recovery. But, it wasn't as if I were evil or bad; I was sick. The kleshas occur all through life, and having this discerning point of view to look at them is helpful.

False Understanding

My sickness told me I was *not* sick, and false understanding, the root of all the kleshas, was in play here. I was living an illusion.

This delusional thinking would have me believe that everything is permanent: I will always feel lost and lonely and be in pain, poor, reviled by my children, and mistrusted by my friends. This condition of the false appearing real is the root of the four other sufferings, and I had them all in spades.

Ego

A false sense of self pervaded my life even before I started drinking. Even though I had this false sense of who I was all through my life, it had a huge influence on my attraction to drugs and alcohol. It was the basis for my codependency in my relationship with my parents—my mother who was drinking and my father who had mental disorders. As with a colicky baby, whatever pain I felt defined me: loneliness, disappointment, fear, and insecurity, as well as joy, anticipation, and attachment. Whatever I felt was going to be felt in that same way forever; in fact, I embodied that feeling. When the periods of pain, dissociation, or fear overwhelmed the positive, I found drugs. Then, that persona, that sense of self, "the druggie," became my whole being. I lost my way from my inner true self for so long that I forgot she even existed.

My ego still steps in the way when I am looking at an activity that is obsessive or a situation that is not manageable by me. Over and over, I come back to the fact that I can only do my own work, and I need to leave the outcome to my higher power.

Attachment/Craving

Another way of thinking of attachment is in terms of a craving, an addiction. This is a timeless suffering, documented in eons of writings.

An addict is completely submerged in one's false self, the part that perceives no consequences, lives for the moment of being high, and is completely self-centered. This active user has forgotten his or her true self, that native goodness once known in secure moments as a child.

We addicts have discovered that we can take or do something that makes us feel "better," making us intoxicated beings. The rush of adrenaline in gambling, the feeling of hope and possibility when purchasing something new, and the feeling of being enveloped in a new love—all of these feelings of pleasure—unhinge the mind. Completely distracted from the requirements of the present moment, we are consumed by craving.

The First Step of recovery invites us to see the unmanageability of a life led and consumed by craving. Ultimately, we accept that we are powerless over our substance or behavior. Understanding the affliction of craving can help one grasp why this has been so hard to accept.

Craving can be stimulated anytime we have a process restriction. Anytime we reduce an activity or find abstinence, we can stimulate the phenomenon of craving. It brings us back to the First Step and our powerlessness over an activity and how unmanageable our life can be. I continue to have cravings and attachments; for example, I went through a process of changing my diet for a period of time. It was difficult. I realized how accustomed I was to certain types of food, frequency of eating, and portion sizes. It was a shock. I thought I ate well, and I do, but this period of food-type elimination cranked up the addict in me. I felt hungry when I wouldn't usually feel hungry, and I had a desire for textures and flavors I didn't usually think about—I was craving food.

Aversion

Avoiding the unpleasant was one of the roots of my using and addictive behaviors. I wanted to be distracted from life. Just as I was attracted to the illusion of a "free" life that using promised, I avoided discomfort and responsibility, even success and love. I felt I didn't deserve the good and I was comfortable with the difficult, but I also wanted, in some strange way, to control my pain. I would stay in a bad situation because I knew what it was like, and I avoided change because I didn't know what that would be like. Taking the First Step meant that I was going to have to challenge this klesha and be comfortable with the discomfort.

I continue to struggle with aversion. I don't like uncomfortable conversations or challenging confrontations. I am still triggered in a physical way around loud, emotive, angry people. I prefer to avoid the situation or flee if I can't divert the person's attention and cool them down. And in the process of working with the elimination diet, I found that by eating and snacking I had been avoiding not only unpleasant feelings, but also boredom and sleepiness.

Fear

This affliction—the fear of death, change, transformation, and the space of nothingness between now and then—pervades all the steps and can prevent one from even taking the step before the steps. As we say in the program, "All we have to do is to change one thing: everything," a concept not easily embraced. Beset again by illusions, I fear I am bringing the old me, the person who used, into a new, sober life.

Recovery is really going back to the essence of me, uncovering and discovering my true self. I am not my actions, my body, or even my thinking mind. The real me is beyond all that rational construct, so the fear of change is genuine and has some basis, feeling like a little death. I actually had to grieve the loss of my using self. Once that process was done, I could embrace my new life and being. This experience has been true for many others in recovery. The sooner we can befriend and accept our spiritual nature, the sooner we can let go of this suffering. The other steps will lead us there.

Fear can still propel me to make certain choices and can rule my decisions. I may continue to fear how others will feel, what people will think of me, and being a failure as well as a success. I have learned to experience the feelings, breathe, let go of my fear, and move on.

Koshas and Step One

The koshas are a way to view your being. Imagine a Russian nesting doll: each layer of our being lies within the others. Each layer is affected by the others, so they are not as discrete as the wood of a nesting doll. Instead, think of the layers as membranes or sheaths. When contemplating the disease of any active addiction, we can see that it affects all our layers.

Physical Layer

All the parts that you can touch as well as those inside the body make up the physical layer. Substances, tobacco, and cutting, for example, are all obvious signs of the physical self being destroyed by addiction. This type of behavior is unmanageable and evidence of our powerlessness.

In early recovery, my physical layer was impaired. I had dental problems, digestive issues, and dermatitis, and it was soon discovered I had cancer. (This was a curable and operable cancer, but had I not sobered up at that exact time, it could have become immeasurably worse.) In later recovery, during times of great physical health, I have damaged my physical layer by overeating or overworking. My body pays the price of any excess and addiction.

Energy Layer

This is the layer—the energetic self—that is our life force. Nourished by food, water, and breath, we may experience this layer as vitality. I tried most often to manage this layer, usually giving myself more energy through my drug taking. Later, in a panic, I might try to use drugs and alcohol to come down, to calm my energy. Manipulating this layer was my definition of manageability, and I would have to change that definition to survive and recover.

I had no idea how to manage my energy in early recovery, and always fought my natural energy levels. I had always used drugs or alcohol to turn up or turn down the volume. I was actually unaware of what my energy level was until I crashed. I had lost the tools to understand how I felt, unless it was extreme.

As I have moved into long-term recovery, being aware of this kosha has been invaluable. I eat more wisely and maintain an attitude of gratitude to keep my nervous system calm and coherent. I maintain a proper level of activity throughout the day and practice proper sleep hygiene for a good night's rest. I know I am slipping in my recovery related to overactivity and work addiction when my energy is not revived after a night's sleep, serving as a warning that I have some unattended manageability issues.

Chakras and Step One

Our chakra system will be out of whack as we enter recovery. Today, I still use the chakras to evaluate whether I am in need of a first-step refresher, whether I need to get back to basics, or whether I have things in my life that are no longer wise to manage on my own.

The imbalance of one chakra has an effect on the balance of the others; therefore, they will all need attention. The foundation of our identity, our relationship with the world, our ability to be aware of and change ourselves, our connection to our higher power, as well as the health of all our physical systems have been affected by our addiction. These are the fields of energy that are governed by each chakra.

Substances had an impact on how I felt about the world, what was important to me in the world, and how I perceived the world. Add to that unhealthy nutritional habits, poor sleeping habits, relationships that were built on falsehoods, support that I had asked for and then misused, and so on, and I had violated the wisdom of the seven energy centers in my body. It was overwhelming. Step One helps break down the enormity of the task ahead and tells us to see what *is* and accept it.

Root Chakra

The root chakra governs our foundation, our survival instincts, and our sense of security. I was wildly out of control and insecure in my active addiction. Looking at the First Step with the perspective of the root chakra, I could see the quantum shift that awaited me.

Early in recovery, I had one of those awakening thoughts, a little flash of understanding: that which helped me live will now kill me. In the past, I had thought about killing myself, and there were mornings when I woke up severely disappointed that I had not died in my sleep. I held a gun to my head at one tragic and desperate time, desiring to end my life. However, this understanding of dying and self was different. I wanted to be sober. I wanted to live. The self I was afraid of killing was not the body or the shell of my existence; it was my inner self, my true self. The root chakra is the seat of security, and I wanted to be secure, trustworthy within myself, and grounded in community with others. I wanted to be safe. These are root chakra issues, and I needed to address them.

Sacral Chakra

Sexuality and creativity lie in the sacral chakra. New recovery is fraught with hypersexuality—the need to connect, to be approved of, to distract one from feelings, and to create excitement that can replace a behavior or substance—and this chakra needs care as well during the First Step. People who are addicted to sex and love have special challenges is this area. Once the dulling mask of active addiction is removed, sexuality can replace the adrenaline rush previously provided by alcohol and/or other drugs.

Gunas and Step One

As we begin to take the steps, we find ourselves in different qualities and states of being. Some of us come to recovery from a dark and heavy state of consciousness. Depending on which drugs we were using or behaviors we had participated in, we could also be hyperactive, without the ability to settle down. We could be in a state of either sluggish tamas or wild rajas.

I used drugs to get through my day and alcohol to bring me down at night. When drinking didn't work, I would add other drugs to get to sleep, even for a few hours. Then I would wake up, take something, get the kids ready, and go to work. Next, I would stop at the store to get some booze on the way home and start the whole cycle again.

I was an up-and-down mess when I walked into recovery. The first few weeks were a rajasic tornado. I was full of excitement and hope, but I didn't know how to channel that energy. I made vast to-do lists, enacted new rules and tasks for my small children, and generally became a whirling dervish of good ideas, plans, and goals that could never be completed in any reasonable time. I was out of integrity with "one day at a time." Then I became tamasic, sluggish, and overwhelmed by the smallest thing. For the next few months, I would cycle between the two. I would be all over the First Step, being a shining light of compliance, or I would be in despair, losing hope that life could be any other way than what it had been.

Now when I am overwhelmed and realize I have a first-step issue on my plate, I use the proper power of rajas to move toward a more balanced state. If I get tied up around the process of changing, I am stuck in that overactive rajasic state. When I begin to use the energy of rajas to change and then settle into being, I have approached the harmonious balance that is sattva. I recognize the dull and sluggish nature of tamas, and then, with a proper amount of activity—a level to match the issues at hand—I make and execute step-by-step plans to address the issue. When I have accomplished that, I feel more in harmony and can experience a moment or two of sattva. I have become more sensitive to the swings of these states of being and take actions to soothe my feelings and modify my reactions.

Putting It All Together

Just know that there is no one way to arrive in recovery, nor is there a wrong way. No matter how much we tried to manage—or withdraw from managing—our lives were unmanageable, and there had to be another way. The steps will lead us there.

By being open to all parts of the First Step, I could find the strength to change one thing in my life at a time. The principle behind Step One is honesty. We have an honest desire to cease our addictive substance use or behavior and discover a whole new horizon. We discover that there is another way to live, one that integrates all levels of our being, balances our chakras, and provides a way to view our life. Yoga will help you dig deeper into this process with such concepts as the kleshas, yamas, niyamas, and gunas.

Pose for Step One: Legs Up the Wall

This pose changes everything. As you elevate your legs, this pose will bring relief to your heart. Your perspective changes, as you can only look up. You are supported all along the back of your body by the ground and the wall. Remaining here, you can feel relief turn into impatience, then morph into acceptance and other feelings. What was comfortable can become uncomfortable, with uncomfortable moving to neutral or pleasant.

During Step One, the idea of admitting you are powerless may be a relief, then a challenge, and then, once again, a relief. So, too, the idea of one's life being unmanageable may offer a moment of confirmation;

then, a feeling of obstinacy may arise. In time, you may release back into acceptance. This pose can feel alternately great and then uncomfortable, and then delicious once again.

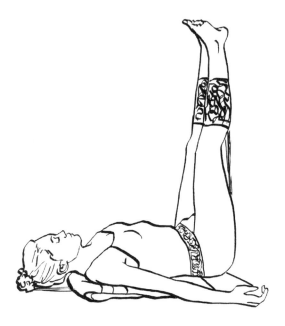

To Come Into the Pose

With a mat or blanket on the floor stretching from the wall into the room, sit on the mat with your right hip against the wall, knees bent, and feet on the floor next to the left edge of your mat (the mat will be behind you). Pivot on your bum, swinging your legs up the wall as you lower your back on the mat. You will hopefully end with your legs up the wall, your buttocks a few inches away from the wall, and your back on the mat. Use a towel, blanket, or cushion behind your head to keep your neck neutrally aligned, with your face parallel to the ceiling. Stay here for five minutes or more.

To Get Out of the Pose

Bend both knees to the chest and pause for a few breaths. Raise your right arm over your head, resting it on the ground. Roll to your right, using your upper arm as a pillow. Pause here again. Use your left arm, then your right, to lever yourself up to a sitting position. Pivot around and lean back against the wall and pause for a few moments.

Grab a notebook or a piece of paper and take a few moments to write about how your body feels after this pose, what your emotional landscape is now, and your understanding of the step. There are no right or wrong answers; this is just a time to make some notes to remind yourself later, if you wish.

"Yoga is the cessation of the misidentification
with the modifications of the mind."

SUTRA 1.2

"When the yogini is firmly established in truthfulness,
she attains the fruits of actions without acting."

SUTRA 2.36

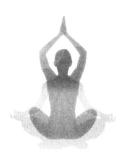

Chapter Two

FINDING COMMUNITY

— STEP TWO —

We came to believe that a Power
greater than ourselves could restore us to sanity.

I was relieved when I read and started working Step Two. I was grateful; I really thought I had been losing my mind. I felt I should be institutionalized or somehow restrained because I couldn't stop using or drinking. I had tried all the tricks: changing liquor types, trying to implement start and stop times, and even taking Antabuse. Nothing helped. In subsequent behaviors that verged on addiction, I felt overcome by the insanity of doing things that I knew were not good for me, such as calling an old flame, eating poorly, or buying something. I was relieved when I discovered I could finally turn over these behaviors.

My drinking and ability to stop had eroded all my confidence. I had proven that I was unable to keep promises to myself or anyone else.

I couldn't make healthy decisions, or if I did, I couldn't keep them. I didn't want to be this slovenly, disrespectful woman with low standards and lower morals. I wanted to be a good mom, a good employee, overall a good person. I entered the rooms of my twelve-step fellowship and heard that it was all possible. I wasn't bad or evil or wrong. I have an illness. Getting well *is* possible, but I realized that I couldn't do it alone. For me, the Second Step was that simple.

That was my faith in the step in its entirety—I could get better, and I couldn't do it alone—until the rebel me got on board when I began to feel better. Then, I took it all back. I started to think I could do it myself, whatever *it* was.

I began to quarrel with the idea of a higher power. I realize now that the Second Step doesn't say anything about a higher power; it just says "a power greater than" myself. As a newly sober and greatly brain-addled person, I knew there were many people who knew better and were doing better than me. I could see that when I looked at the other people in the room with me. However, I was terrified. I didn't want someone to have power over me. I was coming out of a relationship in which someone had power over me, hurt me, and manipulated and harmed my kids. I wasn't about to let someone else take over a position of being in charge of me or my life.

It took some time for me to embrace Step Two. I was being resistant and contrary, but I needed to get that out of my system and cease silly, semantic debates over the words in the step. People in the program suggested I stay open to the ideas and listen to what people had to say at meetings. So, I started to listen. I discovered that the people in the fellowship weren't saying this person or that person had power over them; instead, they talked about how the collective community, the greater wisdom of the group, was a power greater than oneself. That made sense to me, so that was where I started. The community as a whole, and no one individual, could together guide me to health.

I did interpret the word *sanity* as if I were insane, and initially that was the case. I was deranged. I was delusional. I was unable to think clearly and, in many ways, I was unable to take good care of my children and myself. I wanted to be in my right mind, desperately.

I have also thought of the word *sanity* in terms of the French word *santé,* meaning "health." I had lost health in body, mind, and spirit. I wanted to return to emotional health, and I wanted physical and spiritual health as well. I recovered my health slowly with the help and guidance of many people in my fellowship. They had demonstrated the ability to follow a guidance that brought them back to health and shared that wisdom with me. They were showing me how to have appropriate power in my life: not power *over,* just simply power.

In later recovery, I have had occasion to use this step with other behaviors, and the idea of a power greater than myself has had applicability here, too. I looked to the wisdom and support of others when I was letting go of issues such as overspending, overworking, and codependency, in which I tried to manipulate and control others. I could not make the necessary changes alone, and the need to return to sanity was more important than doing it myself. I reached to the steps to heal, and Step Two was critical to the process.

Using Step Two to evaluate the impacts of my behavior on my energy, psyche, sense of self, and spiritual condition was assisted by the teachings of yoga. Specifically, I used tools described in the first chapter. I applied a yogic point of view to the repercussions of my addictions.

Niyamas and Step Two

From the niyamas, or observances, I rediscovered surrender and continued to practice discipline.

Surrender

I surrendered the discussion with my addiction, the "will I or won't I?" conversation. I now realize that whenever I entertain a possibility, I wear down my ability to resist. As they say in the rooms of my fellowship, "If you hang out in a barbershop long enough, eventually you will get a haircut." In other words, if I choose to consistently engage in dialogue or proximity with triggers, lures, or indulgences—whether it is M&Ms or a dating website or sitting on the bar side of a restaurant—I will eventually wear down and try them. My practice is to surrender to my higher power, my wiser authentic self, and walk away. My victory is in leaving, not in staying with a dangerous point of view or temptation or in a dangerous place and trying to be strong.

I learned about surrender and leaving in my first two months of recovery. I was still living with my dealer boyfriend at the time, a chapter in my life I was calling "against all odds." I made up this story that against all odds I was going to remain clean and sober living with people who were drinking, using, and staying up all night. I came to realize that this was a stubbornness that would soon fail. I surrendered by getting out of Dodge and finding a new living situation. I was practicing the observance of ishwara pranidhana and surrendering to a power greater than myself.

Now in later recovery, when revisiting Step Two with the knowledge that health is available to me, I continue to be relieved from anxieties and worry-related discomforts, and I am comforted by the idea that there is a power greater than myself. I am reminded that I no longer have to do it all. I do my best to do my best and then let karma, the consequence of my effort and actions, take it from there.

Discipline

I return to the simplicity of Step Two time and again; it's a matter of discipline. It is a step that I seem to slip or trip on, lose my grip on, and then regrasp. When I discover that I am not feeling sane in a relationship, making frequent purchases, or eating a particular kind of food, I return to Step Two. I go back to basics, practice Step One, and know that in Step Two I can return to sanity. While it is true that it is "practice, not perfection," we also say that it "works if you work it," and work takes discipline.

Kleshas and Step Two

The discussion of Step Two in *Twelve Steps and Twelve Traditions* gives us a few examples of people for whom Step Two may be problematic. They include those who have once had faith and have lost it, those who scoff at faith, and the intellectual, the self-sufficient man or woman.

There is also the defiant one, that person who lives his or her life in defiance of any concept of a higher power—a higher power that has, perhaps, previously disappointed. All of the kleshas are involved in these resistances and rejections.

False Understanding

What do we expect from a higher power, and what do we "count" as the existence of one? Does our higher power have to prove itself directly and immediately? Do I have to see the outcome of Step Two in the next breath? How impatient am I?

This sense of urgent results may be interpreted as a false understanding of what a higher power does in our lives. Little and slow has been the progress of all my authentic growth. On a subtle level, we may have a false understanding of our mind and outlook. We may need to revisit our understanding of the world and bring it back to reality. In recovery, I have learned to look at life a little differently than I had. My prior view of life had been a bit distorted, and a higher power can be my corrective lens.

Ego

When I began Step Two, it was all about me; I could do whatever needed to be done in recovery by myself. This way of thinking—I am separate and have complete dominion over myself to the exclusion of all others—is a mistaken idea. This false perception guided me even in my drinking career when I believed I was the only one affected by my decisions. This was not the case; the illusions of the ego fed this mistaken belief.

This false sense of self, this distorted ego, expanded in my recovery to include a sense of self that was the result of other people's opinions of me. My worth was determined by their approval. This madness snowballed into my overworking and undervaluing my family, my friendships, and my self-engendered self-esteem.

Attachment/Craving

This affliction may influence one's concept of a higher power. We may think that our higher power, if it really exists, is there to give us what we want and provide no discomfort or delay. In the *Twelve Steps and Twelve Traditions* this is described as a Santa Claus God: one who brings us only treats.

Thinking in this manner got me to use in the first place: I was going to feel good all the time, and there would be no worries or discomforts in my life. However, this was not to be. The fallacy of this thinking was evident at the end when there was nothing but worry and discomfort. Learning to view life without the phenomenon of craving is to learn to live without the illusion of a single answer to all life's challenges.

Aversion

I had an aversion to all negative feelings, which turned into avoiding all feelings. My feeling barometer broke. When drinking and using to avoid conflict, pain, anger, frustration, and the experience of abandonment, loneliness, awkwardness, or rejection, I also ended up dulling my feelings of care, happiness, joy, freedom, and companionship. I had dulled them all, the unintended consequence of muting or obscuring the unpleasant or painful.

I avoided responsibility for my actions. I also avoided letting go of responsibility. It was a habit that was difficult to give up in recovery. How was I going to trust a power greater than myself to return me to sanity when I couldn't trust anyone or anything? Certainly, I concluded, I could think my way through this. I used to be a good student. I used to be able to work things out. Maybe I could just find reason, and that would return me to health. I was trying to use the mind that got me into this situation to get me out. As Albert Einstein said, "We can't solve problems by using the same kind of thinking we used when we created them." I could no longer cling to what I knew; I needed a higher power.

Fear

This klesha threatened to stand in the way of my transformation. In spite of the fact that I was ready for a new life, I feared change with all my heart, a fear not unique to me. Change is a discussion topic in many meetings. Along with a new belief system that could "return me to sanity" was the understanding that I couldn't remain as I was. It seems simple and clear, but I was unprepared for the unknown.

Adequate food and rest and normal waking hours were about all I could tolerate in the beginning. I was not sure what sanity would look like, and I wasn't certain I was ready. The kula, or wise company in the rooms, assured me that I only had to take it one day at a time and have a little faith; I would not be led into harm.

Koshas and Step Two

Layers of my being—the koshas—were all impacted by my years-long practice of the bad habits I had formed. My emotional, intellectual, and spiritual sheaths were challenged in the Second Step. I wanted to get better; however, I didn't want to change. My emotions were raw, my intellect was confused, and my spiritual self was just coming online. Both seeing the effect of my addiction on these layers and noticing how awareness of these layers might help me with Step Two was encouraging.

To be clear, I didn't have this lens in early sobriety. I developed it later, in the "teenage years" of my recovery. It is in later use of the Second Step with relationships involving my children, money, my husband, and food that I have used the koshas as a model for understanding and applying this step.

Chakras and Step Two

I found that the root, solar plexus, heart, and crown chakras are the primary chakras involved in understanding and absorbing Step Two. I needed to discover grounding through my root chakra in order to reach for a higher power. Incorporating my sense of self, even tenuous and fleeting, gave me the permission and power to reach for my higher power as I found balance in my solar plexus chakra. Compassion and trust in my heart chakra were needed as I began to evolve. Using the grounding and security I developed with my connection to others and opening my heart to willingness and compassion, I was then, tenuously, able to access and balance my crown, or spiritual, chakra. Having established even an intermittent connection with my crown chakra was going to be critical to move on to Step Three.

Gunas and Step Two

Rajas, or the quality of movability to an appropriate degree, was once again my friend. When stuck in the tamasic state of fear and insecurity, I was unable to change. Mired in old thinking, I was unable to see, much less conceive of, a power that could do for me what I could not do for myself. Indeed, getting sober was something I needed help with.

There were times when the fluctuation of faith would pull me away from believing in a power greater than myself or that there was sanity for me. Excess movement, or rajas, was turning my surrender off and on like a bad fluorescent light. A moderate amount of mutability and ability to change were what I needed. It took work and vigilance to stay in right balance with this state.

Putting It All Together

Contemplating the concepts behind the yogic wisdom, you can find additional ways to look at Step Two and discover what is challenging for you, as well as what you can use to clear away the veils and see with a clearer vision. Sutra 2.2, located at the end of this chapter, combines both discipline and letting go in order to avoid afflictions—mental, physical, and spiritual impurities—and can serve as a Step Two verse. The discipline of referring to your higher power will help bring you back into health at all levels.

Pose for Step Two: Child's Pose

Release your cares. Take a moment and return to sanity—body, mind, and spirit. Looking for comfort in this pose, practice maneuvering yourself around, using props so that there is minimum pressure on your joints (hips and knees particularly). This pose represents a break, a breath, between doing one thing and another. It is a time to resuscitate yourself and come to your senses—all of them—including your thoughts, your view of your thoughts, the sensations in your body, and your views and opinions about how you feel in your body, mind, and spirit. Also called the pose of wisdom, this is a pose that allows us to let it be.

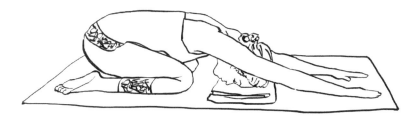

To Come Into the Pose

Kneel on a blanket or soft towel on the mat or floor. Touch your toes together behind you and move your knees apart—about shoulder width or more. Fold forward and bring your head to the ground, either directly or by placing it on another folded towel, block, or your stacked fists. With your head on a form of support, stretch your arms out so that you can be comfortable through your shoulders and back. Get heavy. Breathe. Remain here for three to five minutes.

If being on your knees is difficult, you can put a folded blanket in between the back of your thighs and your calves, tucked in behind the knee bend. If this doesn't work, you can lie on your back close to the wall with bent knees and let the soles of your feet rest on the wall, or lie on your back and put your calves on a couch or a chair. The important thing is to curl up with support and let go.

To Get Out of the Pose

If you are in the traditional child's pose, bring your hands on the floor beneath your shoulders and push down to rise up. Scoot around into a seated position with your legs extended. Take a moment here to reflect. If you are in another arrangement, roll to your side, pause, then pivot around to end in a seated position with your legs extended. Pause and reflect.

Find your notebook and make an entry. Check in with your body, mind, and spirit. What is your relationship with your health and your higher power at this moment?

"The yoga of action (kriya yoga) is practiced to
bring about samadhi [bliss, or union with the divine]
and to minimize the colored thought patterns."

SUTRA 2.2

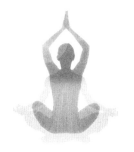

Chapter Three

TURNING IT OVER

— STEP THREE —

We made a decision to turn our will and our lives over
to the care of God *as we understood Him.*

The Twelve Steps are often categorized in three sections: the foundation steps (Steps One through Three), the working steps (Steps Four through Nine), and the maintenance steps (Steps Ten through Twelve). The more grounded we become and completely accept the first three steps, the stronger the infrastructure, which is the bedrock of our recovery.

The last of the foundation steps is Step Three, which both challenges and releases us. We may say, "Yes! I am no longer in charge! Wait, if I'm not, who is?" This step was a blessing and a curse for me because I had made a mess of my life, making all my decisions in light of my addiction. I had no playbook for a sober life. Finding my higher power in the previous step and now referring to it and relying on it were going to be key to a healthy life going forward. Letting go of hurts and pains, plans and expectations, was going to be a big part of that process.

As I continued to work on my recovery, I heard this phrase repeatedly: "That sounds like a third-step issue." Indeed, when I experience something that I have no control over, I have a choice. I can suffer as I try to control or command it, or I can turn it over. But to whom? Yoga maintains that the greatest freedoms come from giving all to "the Lord," to the divine, to the universe. If yoga has a goal, it would be union with the divine.

Step Three challenges us to decide, to let go of control, and to surrender what we cannot do for ourselves to some other entity or being. This, in itself, requires trust. Trust, as a verb, is an action we take, often taking the form of non-action. We don't have to do anything! That is our Third Step. We cease doing, pushing, trying, and striving. We let go.

This letting go is based on faith. I have faith that my higher power will allow the world to continue, as it ought. It will continue in a manner that I wish or in a manner that I don't wish. But, it will continue. That is a hard pill to swallow for this addict. I am sure, until the last possible moment, I can move things to happen the way I wish they would. I want to control the outcome by manipulating the commencement, the beginning and the unfolding.

The myth of having complete control is one that vexes many of us throughout recovery. The self-will that energizes and propels us when we are in our active addiction—when we allow nothing to stand in our way of using—is misguided, but habitual when we step into recovery. In my case, getting sober revealed all my issues as an adult child of an alcoholic. I slipped from my addiction driving the train to having my feelings—the need to control, the fear of abandonment and manipulation, low self-esteem, and being judgmental—jump into the driver's seat, each aspect jockeying for position to be in charge. Later, I would add other self-sabotaging characteristics and self-defeating behavior patterns to the list. And, this was after I got well.

Using the Serenity Prayer, I was able to begin to parse issues: What was out of my control? What is my decision? What could I surrender? This simple guidance helped me break things down, uncurl my fist, and open my hand to an unknown future. I repeatedly clenched my hand again, thinking, "Oh! Not this! Surely I can handle/manage/control this!" And yet, taking the decision back makes it no easier to surrender a third, fourth, or fifth time; in fact, it can be more difficult. In early recovery, I made a habit of turning things over and then grasping them back—usually in the dark of night when I had difficulty sleeping. I would take a problem from earlier in the day and, like a lozenge, roll it around and around in my mind, deciding and redeciding until I thought I would lose my mind.

I knew better, though. I had taken the Third Step before and was willing to turn my will and life over. The moment I clench the fist of self-will around my problems—denying myself access to reliance on and faith in my spiritual connection—is the moment in which I have taken my will and my life back. When I grasp onto the idea that I know what a change or outcome should be, I haven't really turned something over. I may have decided that the present situation cannot stand, but I am holding onto what I think the new situation should be. I had to practice letting go over and over. It took discernment, taking myself back to the yogic advice of "practice, practice all is coming."

In early recovery, I hardly knew when I was relying on self-will. I was just learning to take responsibility, be reliable, show up, and develop routines and structure in my life. I confused these with the idea that I had control. And when events in my perfect plan didn't unfold the way I thought they should, I felt betrayed. If I had left work on time to meet with my kid's teacher and there was an inordinate amount of traffic causing me to be late, I would just about lose my mind. I was nervous. I was anxious, full of excuses, filled with guilt from the past when I hadn't remembered or been too loaded to show up. All that shame drowned out my faith, and I felt forsaken. I put way too much into what the Third Step could and could not do. I was secretly asking for proof— proof that could only be found by having a seamless life where nothing went wrong. I redoubled my reliance on self-will for a time after any of these imagined disappointments.

Focusing on the last part of Step Three, "to the care of God as we understood Him," I would reacquaint myself with my higher power over and over. It was as though I had to re-form and rediscover my higher power each time I reached for it. Once I let my faith falter, once I stopped trusting, it was like starting from scratch. I had to learn to turn it over again and again.

This process occurs not only in the big issues in life, but also in the small ones. Turning it over happens with the outcome of a project and finding a parking place. Neither one is of great consequence to the eternal scheme of things, but my attitude, behavior, and response are of great consequence to those I love and those around me. Over the course of time, I discovered that proof of the existence of my higher power was the result not of getting my way but of my heart being open to whatever way emerged.

In later recovery, as I was able to see the other aspects of my character that I needed to let go, the Third Step helped here, too. When my self-will was governing my actions, I discovered that I was attempting to hold onto outcomes and manage my life accordingly. I was trusting only in myself. When I was feeling less than others—still coming from the self—I started looking for affirmation and acceptance from others. When I was needy, I had no boundaries, and when I felt wronged, I held onto resentments with a passion. When these situations came up, when I was no longer comfortable sitting in the discomfort of self-centeredness, I came back to Step Three, and this gave me comfort. I was, indeed, in the care of something greater than myself, the unity of spirit and the good that were around me. Long into recovery, I still find challenges to my emotional sobriety, and returning to the basics is a way to ground me again.

Step Three is kind of a lighthouse step, a guidepost. It invites us to continually reaffirm, refocus, and realign ourselves with our higher purpose. In Step Three, we set an intention, an intention to live by new, different values and sensibilities that are no longer driven by our incessant need to avoid discomfort and seek an unreasonable amount of pleasure. The beacon of our higher power will show us the way.

In this action step, we make a decision, but this resolution may wither or morph in time. Many people in recovery often say that they decided to hand over their will and life once to a higher power, and that was it. That is not my experience; I can only speak from that. In the past, I had been convinced that I had turned my will and life over to the care of my higher power and yet suffered from grasping onto a situation or outcome. This had been evidenced by the fact that the expressed desire to rely on my higher power somehow slipped despite my best intentions.

Yoga offers several ways to reflect on Step Three. Going back to the component parts—deciding, controlling, and surrender—we can investigate what these mean to us. In addition, we can look at ways we can find our higher power all around us: less self-centered actions and more actions based on ethics.

Yamas and Step Three

Non-attachment asks us to cease grasping, grabbing, and holding. We need to work toward letting go of people, places, and things and how we want our moment, day, and life to work out. The self-will that comes from the misapprehension of the idea of self can cause problems in this area. When I am attached to an outcome, I feel bad. Nothing except that one outcome will suffice. If I give my will and life—the organization and unfolding of my life—to my higher power, what happens is just right. It may not be what I want, but it will be fine.

Niyamas and Step Three

The observances, the niyamas, give us tools to focus ourselves in the process of taking Step Three.

Self-Study

While I don't need to know all the machinations of my mind or all the alternative outcomes, I do make a mental decision, followed by the action of stillness, in turning my life over and letting go to my higher power. Being cautious to avoid the "paralysis of analysis," I open the fist of my mind, changing it to an open, giving hand. Serenity is often the first part of knowing what I release; it is the way to realistically embrace the choice of letting go.

Surrender

This niyama is a third-step prayer in itself. Knowing that I don't know it all is a huge relief. Finding a higher power and maintaining trust in that higher power is a second part to the prayer, the intention. I am limited in my understanding, the clarity of my thinking, my unattached emotional understanding, and the clarity of my memories. This limitation influences the solutions that I see and also seek. My higher power has no such restrictions or boundaries.

Kleshas and Step Three

Mistaking what we see, think, or feel for the totality of our true self is confirming the misperceptions of the ego. The obstacle of the shallow or less evolved part of ourselves takes over. Turning our will and our lives over to our higher power is really turning ourselves over to the deeper and more abiding ethics and values that begin to emerge and unfold during our recovery.

Koshas and Step Three

How can we better connect with our spiritual selves? What preset ideas, prejudices, and vestigial emotions do we need to disconnect from in order to achieve a clear and abiding union with our higher self and our higher power? In Step Three, we seek to bring alignment and energy to the innermost layer of our koshas, the bliss layer.

Chakras and Step Three

The chakras can provide a way to notice how our energies and feelings have become misaligned. They also provide some clues as to what we can focus on to become more balanced in our recovery.

Root Chakra

Working from the ground up to balance our chakras, we start with the root chakra. This chakra is where we hold our belief systems, our grounding, and the information passed to us from our core group, our family. As we transition away from the possibly faulty wisdom of our birth family or the mores of our pals in active addiction, we move toward a new, healthier, normative existence.

This change can shake our core, and we may falter. When our feelings of security are overexpressed, we can feel needy. Perhaps, we will need proof that a higher power exists because we don't have a lot of faith. Or, maybe we are overconfident in our self and find it difficult to let go of control. This, too, is a lack of faith. A steady reliance on our higher power and a confidence in our new values will bring balance to the root chakra.

Solar Plexus Chakra

The center of our self-esteem and self-will, the solar plexus chakra is the nexus of control and competence. Out of balance, it can be exhibited by a controlling nature. In balance, it can provide a sense of healthy self-control. When this chakra is overactive, the confidence we experience is more along the lines of braggadocio rather than a healthy sense of self. When the chakra is underactive, feelings of self-deprecation and lack of worth will be felt. The solar plexus chakra is also the center governing change and transformation. An adequate amount of activity and energy is to be sought. Lethargy prevents us from participating in our own recovery, and an excess of activity will distract us.

An imbalance in the solar plexus chakra may have had a part in active addiction, creating a feeling of less than, not being a part of. Another impact may have been either overinvolvement in activities that diverted our attention from our pain or underinvolvement in life, making us recoil and retreat and feel as though we didn't deserve to belong.

In recovery, an out-of-balance solar plexus chakra certainly contributes to emotional relapse, if not other forms of relapse. When we try to control or retreat, we behave from an over- or underactive solar plexus chakra. Checking in with this chakra will be a useful gauge of how well we are doing with the Third Step.

Crown Chakra

A connection with our higher power is important as we develop our intuitive response to living life on life's terms. When living the life of an active addict, we make life choices primarily in juxtaposition to how a decision would help our continued relationship with our behavior or substance. This type of behavior comes from a *lower* self. However, making decisions in pursuit of a life of recovery comes from a *higher* self. Finding balance in the crown chakra is the pursuit of a life in right relation to one's higher self: no more defining oneself by how bad one can be, but rather by how balanced one can be.

Gunas and Step Three

Mutability moving toward harmony embodies the gunas utilized in Step Three. We need rajasic motion in the action of turning over our will and our life, and the resultant condition is harmony. How do you know if you have turned over your will and your life? You may experience a sense of oneness, of union, with your "fellow man," perhaps a feeling of serenity.

Putting It All Together

Addiction was isolating. All my choices and decisions had been made in reference only to my needs, my pleasures, and myself. Life in recovery is life lived in a broader view, with more of humanity being considered. Consider others in your choices, decisions, and plans. Reflect on and rely on your higher power to work out things that are happening in your life.

Pose for Step Three: Modified Lying Pose with Props

You will need a bolster or rolled bed pillow, a block or thick book, and a blanket or towel. If you have tender shoulders, find two more towels to have handy. If you don't have a bolster, you can make one by folding a medium-firm-to-firm pillow in half. Then, slip two or three rubber bands or some other fastener over the pillow to keep the fold in place.

This modified lying pose supports the back and opens the heart. You are supported by, or put in the care of, the props. To become willing to be cared for, allow yourself to use as many props as you need today and find comfort in the pose. Permit yourself the privilege of testing the waters to see what works. You may think that you don't need towels for your arms, but when you get into the pose and stay there for a while, your shoulders will ache and you will remember that you could have cared for yourself a little better by allowing the props to support you. It happens to us all. Use more than you need, and then move them away if you like. Take a moment to make yourself comfortable again.

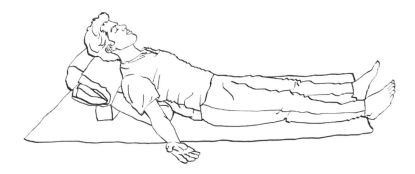

To Come Into the Pose

Place your mat about a foot from the wall so you have plenty of room around you. Set your thick book or yoga block at one end of the mat. Place one end of your bolster on top of the book, with about six inches of it hanging over the top. If you have a dense bolster without much give, you will want to place a towel or blanket across the raised top of the bolster as a pillow for the back of your head.

Sit with your hips a few inches from the base of the bolster and lie back, placing your head on the raised end. You will be lying on essentially a ramp, and your torso will be raised, with your head perhaps a foot from the floor. Extend your legs on the ground. If this is not comfortable for you, bend your knees with the soles of your feet on the floor, or flop the knees out into a butterfly pose with the soles of the feet together. Turn the arms, palms up, out to the side in a T position. Your outstretched arms will be hanging open with your upper arm off the ground and your hand and/or forearm on the ground.

Notice how your shoulders feel. Would you benefit from a towel or blanket under the elbows and forearms? If your shoulders are uncomfortable, move your arms from the T position closer to the hips. You could even put a folded towel underneath each arm to reduce the angle from the shoulder to the ground; bring the ground up to you. Get what you need to be comfortable and then rest here for seven to ten minutes. It takes some time to turn yourself over to the care of another, even in a pose. Give yourself time and notice how you feel at the level of all five koshas.

To Get Out of the Pose

Take it slow. If your knees are not bent with feet flat on the ground, please move to that position. Raise your arms up, reaching the hands toward the ceiling. Bend your elbows, drawing the arms in and rolling to one side as you push yourself to a seated position. Sit there for a few moments. Check in again with all five koshas.

In your notebook or on paper, write down your experience of the pose as well as a few sentences about how you feel at each of the five levels of your being: the physical, energetic, emotional, intellectual, and spiritual layers.

"Samadhi is obtained through
devotion to Isvara (Supreme Being)."

SUTRA 2.45

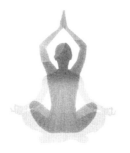

Chapter Four

LOOKING INWARD

— STEP FOUR —

We made a searching and fearless
moral inventory of ourselves.

The Fourth Step is both scary and satisfying. Courage is the quality that is required to embark on this phase of our recovery. With this first of the working steps, there is visible proof of the actions we are taking. We write. We set down on paper the happenings of our life in active addiction or in another period of life we are examining. Our writing becomes an inventory of our moral challenges. It is also a contemplative step: we practice consideration, internal focus, and reaching back into memories. Using discernment, honesty, and courage, we bring the past to mind in a new way—a way that investigates the operational forces behind the choices we have made.

If we are stuck in some area of our life, or feel stagnant or uncomfortable, we may be stalled in our recovery. When the same annoyances, issues, and frustrations appear repeatedly, when we find ourselves doing the waltz—Steps 1-2-3, 1-2-3, 1-2-3—on the same behaviors and attitudes, we may need to move to Step Four. The inertia, depression or aggression, and anger we feel may indicate that there is more work to do. We eventually become too well to tolerate being sick anymore.

The Big Book suggests using the multicolumn format for Step Four. *Twelve Steps and Twelve Traditions* contains further guidance. Narcotics Anonymous and almost all of the other 140-plus recognized anonymous programs offer their approaches to the inventory process. In addition to needing that special pen or pencil and the proper pad of paper, we may also have access to online worksheets. It is tempting to shop around for the perfect supplies and perfect format, thereby delaying the actual work. My sponsor guided me to simply choose one and get started. I would otherwise have been caught up in the process of selecting rather than the process of doing.

Whether for the first or the nth time, two things surface for me: *procrastination* and *perfectionism*. I allow these two qualities to derail my efforts and obscure the truth. The heavy and inert feelings prevented me from proceeding, and the illusion of perfectionism both drove me on and made me feel inadequate in my work. Procrastination would have me write down too little, and perfectionism would have me thinking that whatever I wrote was not enough.

As I work, I also have to avoid blame. My initial try at Step Four was all about *them* and how I had been hurt, angered, abandoned, martyred, or disregarded. Yes, things had been intentionally and unintentionally done to me. From the time I was a child until the day I put the bottle down, I had been in the way of harm. Using the Big Book's examples regarding resentments, fear, and insecurity, for example, I had developed quite a list.

There were times when what happened could not have been predicted, with outcomes for which I was not at fault. On deeper investigation, however, I discovered that most events had resulted from my own bad decisions. Whether the inventory was about my drinking career or my overwork and ego-centered job performance, most of the aftermath was due to choices I had made.

At first I tried to edit as I wrote, finding only those incidents in my life that fell easily into a three-column format: (1) "I am (resentful, fearful, angry, sexually inconsiderate) at ____"; (2) "The Cause"; and (3) "Affects My ____." If I couldn't put it in that grid, I simply avoided the topic.

I was pretty bewildered in my first few years of recovery, as my ability to discern degrees of character flaws and levels of responsibility had been impaired. I was unable to grasp the "nature of [my] wrongs." My sponsor and my therapist helped me to weed through the information to find the harm, the supposed reason for it, and how it had manifested in my life. I listed the picayune and the prodigious; in truth, I had no internal barometer to measure which was which. Even as I became aware of sensate feelings, I had little discernment. The ability to feel was turned either all the way on or completely off. I liken my first Step Four to going through snarled hair with a wide-toothed comb—I got the big tangles out, but there were still knots. I would get those out later as my stability and self-awareness improved.

My hatha yoga practice taught me a similar lesson: hold your poses with the condition of your body at that moment, avoid doing harm by overreaching or overstretching, and stay within your capacity at this time. In recovery, both early on and later, I do what I can. Clearly, my ability wasn't that great in the beginning. What was true, however, was that I had made a complete, honest, and courageous attempt at it.

As I got healthier, my thoughts cleared and my ability to recognize and appreciate subtler, more complex emotions improved. As this happened, new memories resurfaced, and many remembered situations bothered me. I felt more responsible for things that had happened and choices I had made. I eventually needed to go back and revisit Step Four and separate the issues on my inventory into the event, the trigger for the event, and how I responded to the event. The purpose of that step made more sense later, and I was able to use a finer-toothed comb.

You, too, may find that when you are emotionally strong enough, when your self-esteem has risen enough to allow you to feel stable, you may be prepared to see not only how the *acts* of drinking and using had affected others, but also how your values (or lack thereof), such as selfishness, control, and jealousy, and your fear, low self-esteem, and anxieties had damaged others. You may be ready to gain additional insight into the shadow side of yourself—the manipulative actions, the controlling ways, the manifestations of resentments, and the fear. When I became well enough, with my personal ethics more firmly established, I could see my past with wiser eyes and a more compassionate heart. I was well enough to look into my past for the true reasons for my behavior rather than for self-punishing ones.

Once living a sober life, we have an opportunity to look at our relationships, our sexuality, our job, our family, and our finances. When we are less distracted by undefined or overwhelming feelings, our behavior becomes clearer. Taking the time to determine our values and ethics after practicing the principles of the program for a while may lead us to a deeper examination of our past behavior. These forward strides in our recovery may affect how we regard ourselves and perceive our dignity and understanding of the past.

We may discover memories or feelings of anger—not just anger with our self, but anger we had held with others. We may find we had been furious with past circumstances, with society, and with people around us. We may find ourselves outraged with how we have been treated due to our race and assumptions about our gender and our abilities. We may be disappointed with the options we felt we had at times in our lives, the wages we were paid, or feelings of being discounted.

When I reviewed Step Four, I found I *was* angry at society as a whole and with individuals in the ways they had demeaned me. I was angry that I had demeaned myself in pursuit of drugs and alcohol. All these feelings and more came rushing back. I found I had pushed these emotions inward, manifesting in depression, guilt, and shame. As I grappled with these feelings, my sense of self-worth was reduced further. Therefore, it was time to address the sources of my anger and take responsibility for how I expressed it.

We may get in touch with resentments at a new level. We may find a current resentment that needs addressing, and we may also find resentment resurfacing from the past. A friend in long-term recovery discovered resentments at her parents, extended family, sister, and brother. She discovered these at a different level of resentment than the childish feelings she had been able to access in her first go-round through Step Four. At that point, she had simply resented times she didn't get her way or wasn't given money when she had asked for it. This time, she expressed a deeper, more fundamental pain, which included feelings of abandonment, insecurity, deep loneliness, and a longing for the care and safety she thought a child should have and feel. She was resentful about things that would never materialize, and she was making the world pay the price for her loss in false expectations and bitter behavior.

Fear that has been stuffed and denied for years may finally come out. In my case, while working Step Four I realized that some of my risky choices and lack of care about my own safety had come about from unaddressed fear. It seemed counterintuitive, but I actively put myself in danger to prove I wasn't afraid.

Feelings, such as fear, leak all over. They can manifest in having boundaries that are too firm if we fear letting people get to know us. We can have no boundaries at all if we fear offending others or displeasing them. We may be unable to deal with the unacceptable behavior in a relationship for fear of abandonment. Insecurity and low self-esteem were strong drivers in the "nature of [my] wrongs."

When inundated with feelings of low self-worth, another friend in recovery acted in unfair ways with friends and family. She asked for more assurance and attention from them than was reasonable. She felt slighted if things didn't go her way, as if others were discounting her preferences. Others were paying the price for her feelings of discontent. In actuality, she was responsible for the pressure she put on others and the animosity that it engendered. No one could reasonably fill her unending need for attention and reassurance. The more she tried, the worse she felt.

I had a similar experience. While my parents had told me repeatedly, "No one likes someone who wears their heart on their sleeve," I was (and am) tenderhearted. I, like many people who suffer from addiction, feel emotions acutely; for me, a deep physical sensation comes with sensing a feeling. This can appear as a cold clenching in my heart and shoulders, a cramping in my stomach, or simply a clenching of my jaws, holding my face rigid in resistance.

After I worked the steps, this sensitivity would become an attribute when I learned to modulate it; however, in my Fourth Step I needed to look at what effects my untempered feelings were having on others around me. I would feel deeply, then something small would become drama, my happiness would become hysteria, and my sympathies could smother. I had no dimmer switch on empathy, and it could be exhausting for everyone involved.

Stealing and deceitfulness to get drugs and booze were actions I was able to admit to pretty easily during my first time through Step Four. However, other actions in my using years were not directly related to getting supplies or being loaded; lying and stealing had leaked over into other parts of my life. I had been misrepresenting and prevaricating about things small and large, stealing for justified and unjustifiable reasons. Even in my first two years of recovery, I would still take things that weren't mine and lie for seemingly no reason at all. Making restitution was certainly required, but delving down into the reasons for doing these things was just as important. These unwise actions pulled at my heart and impaired my relationships with others. They demeaned me and disparaged my relationships, and this had the potential to damage our future together and individually. More work needed to be done.

We are told in recovery that feelings are not facts, but I found little comfort in those words. The situations I was recalling were real, the violations of my basic principles were real, and the torment I experienced felt real. Thank goodness for people in the rooms of recovery, because I got to hear my story coming from their lips as they shared their journeys. I heard not only the events, but also their outcomes. My peers had worked through their feelings using the steps and had reconciled with their pasts—proof of the effectiveness of this twelve-step work. They had completed Steps Four and Five, processes that allowed the pus of the past to be expelled so true healing could occur. I trusted that process because I saw it happen for them.

Many people experience further relief from a second or third time through the steps, and I have followed suit. Yoga has given me additional ways to look at my past and more tools to use in healing. I have a greater understanding of what the past is telling me, why I made my decisions, and how best to release the past and re-form my future.

Kleshas and Step Four

One challenge during the Fourth Step is to look beyond the chains of the kleshas; after all, they are obstacles. As outlined in in the sutras, the kleshas offer one way of examining the nature, or driving force, behind our actions and misdeeds. Using the kleshas, we can see how fear, ego, attachment, and aversion appear in our lives and what false perceptions guide our actions.

False Understanding

Avidya can provide a lens through which to look at so many past assumptions and hurts. When others were angry, we may have believed that we were a person who inspired anger. If often criticized, we may have felt that we were wrong, that our work and actions could please no one. When corrected at every turn, we may have felt incompetent. The input of a few pivotal people framed our way of looking at all people, seeing those isolated situations as true for everyone, all the time. These are the ways the unreal can be mistaken for the real.

Thinking that the impure was pure was more easily discerned during my first Fourth Step. I had thought my drinking and using were a personal choice and no one else was harmed—if I could even believe that using and drinking were harmful at all. LSD was the gateway to higher consciousness, and what could be purer than that? I felt more creative when I was high, and I believed creativity was close to spirituality.

In my early days of active use, I was very generous. I wanted a big party around me. Going into debt and risking my kids' food and shelter, I would use my last dime to keep the party going. Again, I was mistaking something reckless as being something fun. I suffered from a profound misapprehension of the world around me. I believed everyone was doing it, no one was getting hurt, and, in my later days when I could barely leave the house, I was sure no one knew the depth of my disease. I was deluded, misinformed, and oblivious. This lack of perception was dangerous to me and others, but my denial was strong.

Later in my recovery, when I became subsumed with my work, I fell prey to the same misunderstandings of the world around me. I thought I was handling everything well and I was good at my job, efficient at home, and completely attentive in all my relationships. That thinking turned out to be false. While I was effective at work, efficiency at home had turned to dogmatism, and I was distracted in everything that I was doing. I was not present with my family and friends.

When we have a false understanding, we can confuse pain with pleasure. That sounds strange; however, there can be comfort in the known and fear about the unknown. In those last years of active addiction, when the fun had long since left and the grasping toward the good old times was a strong draw, a friend of mine was miserable. She knew she wasn't experiencing the pleasure she sought from using, each day trying once again to recapture the illusion of fun, peace, and romance—all the experiences she had partaken in at one time or another, years ago. Hurting herself in body, mind, and spirit with no regard for long-term survival, she drank and used drugs one day at a time, to get herself through the day "just once more."

Later, working through Step Four, she discovered that she had learned to disregard her own feelings: feelings of exhaustion, feelings of physical pain, even an awareness of her need for comfort and support. At work, she was letting her bosses' appreciation—from which she derived pleasure—override her needs. She wouldn't rest when sick or take proper breaks at work; in fact, she even came to work when her kids were sick—just to prove how indispensable she was. A justification for her chronic colds and joint pain was that they were the result of her overworking. It was difficult to give up the accolades in order to care for herself. Her Fourth Step showed her the consequences of ignoring her body.

Ego

How can we separate the image of ourselves we are invested in, the one we want to portray, the self we imagine ourselves to be, from the essence or deep truth of who we are? While drinking or using, we operate under the illusion that we are funny, sexy, or an expert in whatever is going on at the time; however, deep inside, we are berating ourselves for being a liar, unworthy, or a sham. Neither is strictly true, but in the black-and-white thinking of addiction, we are all or nothing.

This black-and-white thinking is not easy to shake, and it follows us into recovery. We don't know who we are without a role or a part to play. While we hear that what others think of us is none of our business, it may take years to learn what we think of ourselves, and even longer to understand that this thinking is merely an aspect of ourselves and not the full picture, or the exact reality of our being.

Using the principle of false ego identification as a guide, you may be able to look at how your actions emanate from your self-image and how to find a truer image of yourself. It took me years to come to the yogic understanding of Sat Nam: "I am truth," or, simply, "I am."

Attachment/Craving

Underneath addiction is deep longing—for recognition, for being seen, for being accepted, for security—for *love*. We wanted to find trust and be trustworthy. We wanted to be close to others and find intimacy. We may have felt a pit of unmet needs inside and had to fill it in a visceral way.

These deeper needs developed into cravings, cravings that were only satisfied with that special person, the right cocktail of substances, or being carried away by feelings, emotions, and pleasurable situations. The Fourth Step can reveal manipulative behavior, a controlling nature, values that had been violated, and the people who had been hurt. This can come in early recovery when we examine our years of active addiction. We can discover how our actions had stemmed from our desire for more: more drugs, more attention, or more stuff. Later, when we have some perspective on the disease of "more," we can catch its symptoms earlier when our behavior reveals the resurgence of craving. We face the reality of these excesses and how they manifested in our desire to satisfy our cravings.

In recovery, we refer to three things that can throw us off of our recovery path: discomfort or disillusionment with *people,* with *places,* and with *things.* Any one of these three can be a source of addiction, and thus can be associated with cravings and triggers. In other words, we develop attachments to people, places, and things.

A friend, working through her steps again at ten years clean, came face to face with the fact that she had an intense craving and attachment to feeling competent, desirable, and respected. She was convinced that the resource for those feelings was outside herself. She wanted to feel calm and serene and thought that a certain job and the perfect relationship would give her what she desired. She kept finding dissatisfaction with her employer and changed jobs and careers. When she was discontented, she found blame in others. She looked outside herself for support and sustenance—her or him, that thing or this place—and this something outside herself was going to make her feel better.

In working Step Four, she was able to uncover some of the sources of her needs, some reasons she kept grasping onto others. Respect came from self-respect; competence came from losing self-doubt and finding the training she needed to develop her authority. She found strength in order to handle the times she felt rocky. The longings for safety, respect, security, and other life assurances have not left her; she has simply found other ways to express her needs. She has also found more ways to resource into her own self. When needed, she can now reach out and collaborate with her universal spirit to supply her with more recognition and support.

Aversion

We don't want to experience pain or feel hurt or disappointment. We don't want to experience loss or uncertainty. We don't want things to be hard. Yet, much of life is made up of these qualities. To grow, you have to change, and in order to change, you have to move through discomfort to something new. It takes effort. It also takes effort to hold onto old ways and ideas when they no longer work, or people and places from the past. It is erroneous to imagine that we could be a new person in recovery and still be as we used to be.

Addiction is the ultimate embodiment of aversion to pain. We use or behave in unhealthy ways to avoid the pain of loneliness, isolation, and abandonment. As a teenager, I was able to transport myself away from the confusion and chaos of my home environment by using or drinking. As an adult, I was able, in the beginning, to avoid feelings of guilt, shame, and despair over my living conditions, my social and employment choices, and my loss of dignity. Avoidance is a driver in so many decisions, and we discover when and how as we work the Fourth Step at any point in our recovery.

The trick to letting go of aversion is to let the energy of discomfort flow. We shouldn't resist or avoid it. We let the difficult feelings be and let them embrace us and then dissipate. Like the physical discomfort of a pose, it passes. There is no always; we won't always feel any certain way. When experiencing the obstacle of aversion, I remind myself that there is no permanent change without pain. If I can reassure and nourish myself in healthy ways, I can face this change and grow—without avoidance taking over and squelching my improvement.

Fear

In early recovery, many of us are paralyzed by thoughts of change. For some, this can be so severe that we experience panic attacks. If we have come from a dysfunctional family, we may have an overwhelming need to know what is going to happen next. We may want to plan how we are going feel about it before it occurs. Sometimes, we have to be in recovery for a while before we become unaware of these processes. They are part of the impact of having grown up in a flawed or maladjusted home.

Fear of change can affect our treatment of others; we stay in jobs or relationships far past their sell-by date, or we avoid jobs or relationships entirely. Eventually, the terror of repeating the unhealthy and damaging known becomes greater than the fear of trying something new, and we "let go absolutely." In my case, I needed outside help. I found a therapist who was able to weave her work with me in and around my twelve-step program so that my healing was a coordinated effort between them both.

If these fears, such as the fear due to a job or location change, the declining health of a parent or other loved one, or the challenge of trying something new, go unaddressed using the tools I now have, all through my recovery I can relapse to old ways of thinking and behaving, ultimately to be mined in another Fourth Step.

To transcend fear, we can use yoga: the breath, the meditation, the poses, and the teachings of the sages. When grounded, we can embrace change for the grace it is. We will be able to meet the sadness of death, the passing of people we love, with an open heart. In feeling the pain of loss completely, allowing ourselves the time to experience the grief in whatever form it takes will allow that adaptation to be authentic and complete. That is a huge gift. Letting go of the fear of death and the fear of change allows us to meet each day as it comes—really living one day at a time.

Koshas and Step Four

Introspection in Step Four can be evaluated on all five levels of our being. Doing the Fourth Step from the perspective of how the koshas have been affected gives you another perspective on the effects of our behavior on ourselves. Perhaps, the disregard for and imbalance in the koshas contributed to some addictive behaviors. This point of view gives us another way to assess the harms we have done ourselves and to discern the type of amends we may need to make later.

Physical Layer

We can use drugs to manage physical sensations. I have a bad back; drugs can help. I feel sick; drugs can help. I have a nervous condition; drugs can help. I am depressed, tired, or bored; food, caffeine, screen time, or cigarettes can help. Pretty soon, whatever I am feeling has one simple solution: deadening feelings with ingestion of substances. Recovery necessitates learning new tools to deal with all these situations. Without these tools, we can continue to do our body some serious harm and threaten our long-term recovery as well. The body and all its systems bear the scars of our life. I was a garbage pail, and my physical body wore the sequelae. I will owe my physical body amends for my whole life.

Unprocessed emotions are trapped in our nervous system and in our muscles. Without care, we can experience chronic conditions such as respiratory problems, immune system disorders, and continuous muscle-tension pain. There are also the long-term viral illnesses that were prevalent in the 1970s and 1980s—and some that are prevalent now. In substance recovery, we can move into sexual behavior that is risky and end up with any of a number of long-term conditions that are difficult to heal.

Energy Layer

Alcohol and other drugs can provide a way to manage energetic needs; so can gambling, accessing porn, or any other brain-altering behavior. The energy layer gets impacted negatively through the addiction process. It will still hold the shadows of the old behavior as well as the imprudent behavior we may indulge in during recovery.

We may find that our energy layer responds to the energy of others—for example, sad when they are sad or feisty when they are feisty. The influence from others' choices, mental states, and situations may move us, and sometimes may overpower us. How have you been susceptible to the energetic influences of others? How do you disregard or override your own energetic needs? Do you rest when tired? Eat when hungry? Use this koshic lens as a tool when taking your inventory.

Mental/Emotional Layer

The information from the outside world comes into us through the emotions and the intellect. The intellect is made up of mental impressions based on our experiences and memories. This is how we see the world. Our experiences growing up, the era and society of our adolescence, and the emotions we felt and those we repressed all have had an indelible impact on this layer of our being. This layer then becomes the filter for what we see and hear.

With a flawed filter or lens, we could do nothing but see in a flawed way: grasping for pleasure and avoiding pain, developing an ego-self that was more rooted in what others thought than in our own values and ethics, and believing the false was real. This skewed mental/emotional layer can cause ongoing issues such as being quick to find fault in others, or finding fault continually in ourselves. We can become suspicious and distrustful, particularly if we are unreliable and untrustworthy ourselves. Prejudices rather than discernments, opinions rather than evaluations, and fears rather than investigation may be the result of impressions made on this kosha. The Fourth Step can help uncover these flaws.

It took much practice to alter my faulty understandings in these states of being. Being vigilant about repatterning my self-talk to be more positive, investigating prior to feeling contempt, and pausing and reflecting before choosing and deciding have all become new, learned behaviors. As a result of this inventory, I pursue friendships with people who are living more estimable lives. I avoid lying, stealing, and harming others and myself. Leading a more ethical life heals this mental/emotional layer.

Wisdom Layer

This layer is the observer, the part that sees us seeing and witnessing what we think and do. The wisdom layer is the center of our character. As we develop new values and redeem old ones, we look into the past to see how we have overridden them in pursuit of self-will.

Hitting doldrums in recovery can be difficult and painful. The joy of growing has dimmed, and the ennui of an everyday life may be stifling. This condition may not be as painful as when we first get clean—the confusion and newness of recovery can be frightening. At that point, there is a clear conflict between how we want to be and how we are behaving.

The sheer banality of the midrecovery plateau can be as dangerous; it sneaks up on us. Meetings don't seem as important, and we may feel we don't have something immediate to offer the newcomer. Who can believe that someone who has double-digit sobriety can understand the feelings and challenges facing the newcomer of today? With disconnection from others, we fall into a dangerous space. It sounds strange, but we can relapse from feeling bored. I have spoken with a few people who were able to come back. They shared a similar story of feeling cured, disconnected, and disassociated. They felt stuck. They stopped doing what they needed to do to stay sober, and they came back as newcomers. If we take the time during Step Four to honor this feeling, we can investigate it. When this dull feeling is bothersome, we can look at it as an opportunity for another awakening rather than relapse.

If our wisdom layer is not integrated with our actions, our character and wisdom are in conflict. When we do our inventory, we can determine how this "care-less" attitude has negatively impacted our lives. It is at this time that a little flicker of faith still burns, letting us know that things can change, that life can be different once again. I believe it was this layer of the koshas whispering to the ultimate layer—the spiritual, joyful, blissful part of myself—that led me to a new moment of grace.

Spiritual Layer

Active addiction can obscure but not kill the spiritual layer of ourselves. As we say in the rooms, we have *done* bad; we *are not* bad. Our spiritual layer is there, patiently waiting to be rediscovered and nurtured. And, it will nurture us in return. I have not found a single moral failing that was driven by this aspect of being. This layer is pure bliss, and actions in recovery are a living amends to this connection to our inner being and higher power.

Yamas and Step Four

We can use the yamas as a road map to investigate the past. They offer us restraints, so we can have healthier relationships with others. Each yama provided an aspect of the harms I had done to others and myself. Using these concepts can help us evaluate and inventory our past.

Non-harming

How have we hurt ourselves and others with words and actions, as well as thoughts? We often forget that harms may come from a lack of action as well. What have we said, done, or thought that was harmful? What did we *not* say or do that resulted in harm?

Non-lying

We may lie, even in recovery, to ourselves and to others. We can convince ourselves of non-truths, and we may have spoken white lies. Investigating the patterns of whom we lied to, why we lied, and what we lied about can give us insight into to the attributes and characteristics of our wrongdoings.

Non-stealing

When using or practicing our addiction, as well in recovery, we may have stolen time, things, care, and honor. We may steal time and objects from others, and time and opportunity from ourselves. In revisiting the Fourth Step and analyzing our actions and inactions, we can evaluate this yama from the perspective of both an addict and a codependent.

Non-excess

Active addiction is excess in and of itself. It can morph into the "disease of more" in recovery with different substances, actions, and triggers. Looking further into our choices and activities, we may be able to see how we had reached for more and more of everything: attention, love, appreciation, and affirmation.

Non-attachment

Clinging, clutching, and needing were all symptoms of my illness. They remained symptoms until the underlying issues were addressed. Until then, they would not go away. I could not let go of self-will, my desires, and my need to have things my way. Until I unearthed the reasons for my fear of chaos and change, I could not address my need to control.

Attachment was the way I viewed the world. Additionally, I made decisions based on "let me get mine first" rather than from a place of abundance, and I never believed that there would be enough for all. I was raised with a sense of deficiency and need, so learning the inherent abundance of life was a journey. During Step Four, we need to take a look at our continued grasping or attachment in recovery.

Niyamas and Step Four

The niyamas give us tools with which to reflect on ourselves and practice introspection and healing. We can use the information from our inventory and allow it to make room for the growth that can occur with a fearless and complete review of our past.

Cleanliness

By doing the Fourth Step, we clean house. Evaluating actions by their motivations and drivers, we can dig deep into our patterns of behavior. Afterward, we may begin to chart a course for a better life with clean motives and a healthy perspective.

Discipline

Particularly in later recovery, we may be tempted to skip Step Four. Considering that we may have had a robust, ongoing tenth-step practice, we may think it unnecessary. However, it is the accumulation of unwise actions that can reveal a theme. The Fourth Step, which can be seen as a compendium of behaviors, can reveal what the theme is rather than having us think that issues are just a one-off. Once we established willingness, the gates opened, and we moved into action. With action complete, transformation can occur.

Self-Study

This niyama is the crux of Step Four. By looking inward and consulting texts such as the Big Book, the *Twelve Steps and Twelve Traditions,* the Basic Text, and other writings, we can begin our journey. In later recovery, I used resources specifically for adult children of alcoholics and gender-specific workbooks. I then referred to the *Yoga Sutras of Patanjali* and the *Bhagavad Gita* in various translations and commentaries to expand my growth. From step-study meetings to meetings with friends and sponsors, we can take healthy direction to reflect on our past.

Chakras and Step Four

The chakras give an energetic framework to evaluate aspects of ourselves. Choices in life may have unbalanced a chakra, or they could have been the result of that chakra being out of balance, or both. Posing questions and considering feelings at these seven levels may enlighten you about how these chakras influenced you. Working with all the chakras, particularly the heart chakra, is useful when inventorying chaotic emotions.

Root Chakra

Looking at balance in the root chakra, which is the source of our security, can help determine what function fear has had in our life. How has our past affected our sense of security? How has our behavior affected the security of others? How do we behave when our security is threatened? When the root chakra is overactive, we may experience hyperactivity, physical aggressiveness, impulsiveness, obsessive sexuality, recklessness, or impulsive behavior. If the root chakra is underactive, we may become manipulative, possessive, overly tired, aggressive, needy, approval seeking, or overly cautious. Does your Fourth Step reveal any of these?

Sacral Chakra

In this seat of emotions and intimacy, we store our feelings. Energy is designed to move, and when we stuff our feelings, we suffer. A state of overactivity, or an overdramatic expression of this energy, can also be destructive, so we look for a happy medium, which can be hard to find for addicts.

If the root chakra is overactive, we may grasp for power or importance, behave selfishly, or become arrogant. We may act overly proud. If this chakra is underactive, we may behave in an antisocial way, become mistrustful, and be unable to express emotions, or we may do the opposite and become an acolyte, a follower. Looking at these questions can provide a renewed perspective on the choices we have made.

Solar Plexus Chakra

We can find the right amount of self-confidence when the solar plexus chakra is in balance. When it is overactive, we can feel judgmental, stubborn, and critical, and/or we can crave constant change. When the energy is blocked, we may feel aloof, be unable to learn, crave recognition, and/or experience feelings of isolation. We may develop psychosomatic problems. When did your lack of self-confidence cause you to lean on others? When did an overage of pride make you boastful or pompous? Look at the fourth-step list with these concepts to learn a little more about yourself, and begin to note these with compassion.

Heart Chakra

This seat of our love, empathy, and joy relates to the flow of emotions. While the sacral chakra also channels love, that love is mainly directed inward. In the heart chakra, the heart moves love up to a higher plane where we can relate to others and the universe. If the heart chakra is overactive, we may find jealousy, stingy attitudes, feelings of being taken advantage of, anger, and overconfidence rather than an excess of sweet feelings and brotherly love. The symptoms of an underactive heart chakra are lack of compassion, need for constant confirmation of self-worth, possessiveness, or a feeling of being unloved. When have you been demanding with your affection? When have you had expectations or been withholding? Note these situations and know that when we find balance in the heart chakra, we can return to joy, compassion, and feelings of healthy, universal love.

Our inventory may reveal that we need confirmation of self-worth and may have done anything to gain approval and acceptance. We have that strange combination of knowing the value of being compassionate and open and having a deep fear of being unlovable, which is a difficult conundrum to pull off—loving others so much that we have little residual capacity for self-love.

The nature of this misguided energy may be revealed in the Fourth Step. The heart chakra can fluctuate between overactivity and underactivity, and our energy may be blocked and stagnant or overactive and uncontrolled. Investigation into how this may have affected our relationships with others can be crucial to understanding the meaning of the fourth-step inventory and our eventual healing.

Throat Chakra

The seat of our self-expression sits in the throat chakra. Holding back our truth can lead to guilt, shame, and blame. An overactive throat chakra can manifest in us as domineering, where we behave in a hyperactive manner or fanatically. The opposite characteristics— resistance to change, stubbornness, and slowness of response to others—occur when this chakra is underactive.

We may find that we can be both bossy and unable to state our needs clearly. We tell people what to do at the same time that we find difficulty in asking for help, support, or attention in a direct manner. We may not be able to express our own truth. It takes time to determine our needs and to express them in a kind way. Our inventory can show us the outcome when this skill is lacking.

Third Eye Chakra

We reflect internally about what we hear, see, and experience. We also connect with our higher power and consider what our internal understanding is. If the third eye chakra is overstimulated, we may express fearfulness, impatience, and oversensitivity. We may also belittle the behavior of others. There is a joke in recovery that states, "I can take anyone's inventory but my own," meaning that we can have a lot of opinions about others, even insight into their behavior, and yet lack that ability for ourselves. If the energy in the third eye chakra is blocked, it can manifest in having difficulty looking inward. We may also experience self-doubt, envy, superstition, action based on fear, and unfounded worries.

I was a worrywart. Constantly anxious, I tried to figure out plans and options for plans, so I would know what was going to happen next and thereby try to control things. These tendencies were revealed in my inventory and appeared in my Sixth and Seventh Steps as some of my shortcomings. I was also one of those people who suffered from the "paralysis of analysis." I became mired in considering all the angles and outcomes of a situation, unable to make decisions. It had affected my family and friendships. Trying to think things through can become a stultifying activity that prevents right action. It can also manifest as overplanning, leaving no room for others' choices or spontaneity.

Crown Chakra

We develop our relationship with our higher power and higher consciousness in the crown chakra, the seat of our spiritual energy. Even this area can be affected by overexpressed or underexpressed energies. When it is overstimulated, we may have an overactive sexual imagination (internal focus), a need to feel indispensable, and a need for sympathy. When the crown chakra is underenergetic, we feel misunderstood, have a negative self-image, lack tenderness to self and others, or are in denial about any number of issues. It is very difficult for crown chakra energy to be in balance when the other chakras are either overactive or underactive.

Our fourth-step inventory may reveal situations that could have benefited from a stronger relationship with our higher power. Tapping into this relationship may enable us to do a fearless Step Four.

Gunas and Step Four

We seek the sattvic state: a place of complete harmony—not too active, not too still. Through drugs and alcohol, we pursued the illusory nature of harmony to the gates of hell. What we found instead was a life of hyperactivity, going nowhere, or tamasic sedentary depression. We looked to people, places, and things to give us contentment; we tried controlling, whimpering, manipulating, and forcing—nothing could satisfy our needs. A fourth-step inventory can help us see what we have been seeking and how we behaved when disappointed.

Putting It All Together

Assessing my Fourth Step and my behavior using these yogic concepts has given me a deeper understanding of myself. I have also discovered that the active use of these yogic tools can give me a long-term way of processing the information discovered during my inventory, which has given me hope that change is possible. This can be possible for you as well.

Pose for Step Four: Supported Forward Fold

Have the same props handy—the bolster, the blankets, and the books or blocks—that you had in the Step Three pose. Have a notebook by your side for writing after you come out of the pose.

Forward folds are soothing and inward-looking poses. It is difficult to learn or do any sort of introspection when we are tense or troubled. This forward fold can calm the mind and loosen the kinks that may prevent honest introspection and discourse.

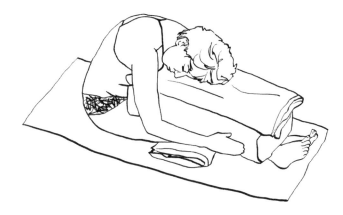

To Come Into the Pose

Sit on the floor with your legs extended; the bolster, blankets, and books or blocks should be nearby. Put one loosely rolled towel behind your knees to keep them supported and slightly bent, in a microbend. Pile the bolster, book, or blocks on your lap covered with a blanket—you don't want harsh edges by your face. Lean forward over the pile. Remove any supports that aren't needed, or add more if you like.

With your knees held in the microbend, let your back round forward with the least amount of effort. Support your head if you like on the bolster or blankets, or let it dangle freely. Let your arms cuddle the bolster or reach forward and hold your ankles or feet. Release intentional gripping of the muscles. Remain here five to ten minutes. Let your breath be smooth and even. Watch your thoughts without becoming attached to any particular idea. Let your brain breathe.

To Get Out of the Pose

Put your hands on the ground next to each side of your body, and walk yourself upright. Put your hands on the ground behind you like a kickstand and stretch, arching your back and looking up to the ceiling. Release. Then back up to the wall for support or gently move to another seated position, so you can write for ten to fifteen minutes about what your thoughts had been.

"Through self-study comes union with
one's chosen deity."
SUTRA 2.44

"As this new wisdom insight strengthens, all previous
mental impressions (samskara) are left behind and the
formation of other latent samskara is obstructed."
SUTRA 1.50

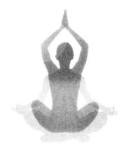

Chapter Five

ROOTING DOWN BEFORE REACHING OUT

— STEP FIVE —

We admitted to God, to ourselves, and to another
human being the exact nature of our wrongs.

This step is going to be scary: sharing your past, the nature of your wrongs, written on scattered pieces of paper or documented in a book or diary. Sharing your vulnerability can be terrifying. While I dreaded reading my Fourth Step with my sponsor, I had also heard that taking Step Five was a great relief. I was conflicted. I didn't want to let someone know everything I had done, and yet I wanted the comfort of unburdening myself. At the same time, I was worried about being judged.

In making my lists about my fears, resentments, sexual misconduct, and so on, I had become aware of events I had forgotten. I could barely believe I had been so mean and crass with others. Yet, I felt I deserved the meanness and crassness I had put upon myself. My first time through the steps, I had still been mired in blame of others for my predicaments, which resulted in my seemingly limitless list of resentments. I was fearful and found no comfort. I was insecure and found no support. I needed love and found that I was unlovable, and I befriended people incapable of loving me. I blamed myself and I blamed others. There was always someone at fault.

According to author T. A. Webb, "A burden shared is a burden halved." Letting go of my secrets and my shames, then as well as now, is a huge step on the path to recovery. Just as my best isn't better than all, my worst is evidently not the worst of all, either. It feels that way when I bottle it up, though, and letting it out reduces the pressure and lightens my load.

My sponsor guided me back to the purpose of Step Five. She suggested that rather than finding blame, I should tell the story and write down the events like a reporter without expressing an opinion or coming to a conclusion. This process worked a little better, and I could look at events from a distance. I was also advised to avoid looking ahead to Steps Eight and Nine, where we would list the people we had harmed and make direct amends where possible. I realized that my fear of the future had gummed up the present—first things first.

My sponsor was kind and allowed me to range freely through my exposition on the first iteration of my Fourth Step. Even though I was stuck in blame, she listened until I was done. She then asked kindly, "Can you tell me about your part in these events?"

I was floored. "*My* part?" I exclaimed. "Surely you can see that *they* were at fault, and I wouldn't have had to do what I did unless they had done what they did!" Clearly, I needed to head back to Step Four, and back to the process. This was a fearless and thorough moral inventory of *my* assets and liabilities, not theirs.

I returned to my task and then returned to my sponsor. I was afraid she wouldn't like me anymore. I was filled with self-recriminations. I felt ashamed and apologetic for everything in my life. Now, I had fallen to the other side of the line; everything was now *my* fault—again, the extreme.

Rather than doing a simple accounting, I added judgment to the mix: I totally lacked moral character and my misconduct was thoroughly of my own making. With a soft smile, my sponsor sent me back to work and asked me to remove words associated with blame and fault before we met again.

After removing conclusions about who was to blame, I returned with an inventory—a document we could work with. By having revisited the issues several times in the rewrites, I had a better idea about what I was trying to achieve in this exercise. I needed to outline how I had acted and reacted when angry, lonely, tired, resentful, fearful, and so on. This work was also leading me to see whom I had lashed out at, whom I had harmed, and specifically what the harm was. This would be good information to lead me to the rest of the steps.

By this point, I had overcome my fear of talking to my sponsor. Reviewing and returning to my work had helped my feelings of anxiety dissipate, and my reaction to meeting with her become more neutral. She hadn't rejected me; in fact, she was inviting me back, time and time again. I was growing to trust her and our relationship. This was a big step for me, as trust was a rare commodity in my makeup at that time.

I also became a part of the people in recovery who had completed the first four steps. I had managed some hurdles in recovery that, if avoided, could have been the gateway to relapse. Many people have relapsed in the middle of their Fourth Step or at the point where they would share in their Fifth Step. I had persevered. I began to feel like part of the herd. We often hear, "Stay in the middle of the herd," as the outliers are prone to drinking or using again. So, I was safe now. I had a community. An expansion of this community occurred when I, in turn, was able to listen to another woman as she did her Fifth Step. This is how we expand the community of recovery: one person supporting another through a common system of healing.

Later in recovery, I was more skilled at doing my Fourth Step and required fewer do-overs with my sponsor. From time to time, I was urged to change my focus—the gift of working with a sponsor—to find a new perspective on my memories, thoughts, and behaviors.

Finding a teacher, or teachers, is as key to practicing yoga as it is to being in recovery. However, I am not referring to pose instructors—although that is important—but to teachers who share the wisdom of the ancient texts, who discuss the concepts and challenge us in our understanding. I have had several of these teachers over the course of my yoga journey. Each person has given me nuggets of wisdom with which to look inward while I connect outward.

Koshas and Step Five

I prepare myself before sharing Step Five. Self-care is a fundamental tool to use before, during, and after sharing this step with another person. Looking at the state of the koshas can help us prepare ourselves for the vulnerability we experience when revealing the discovered truths about ourselves to another person.

Physical Layer

How are you doing physically? Are you getting over a cold or suffering from allergies? Do you have headaches or other aches and pains? Have you exercised lately? Have you taken a walk or practiced some yoga? Is your diet balanced and healthy? Do you have problems with digestion? Discomfort or inattention in any of these areas could throw us off balance and make discussing difficult issues more challenging. I made certain that I was neither hungry nor tired when I went to see my sponsor. I wanted to be present with all my faculties intact.

Energy Layer

Check in with your energy. Do you feel constricted in any way? Are your breath and heartbeat steady? When I went to see my sponsor for this last go-round through the steps, I discovered how important this type of self-care was. I sat in my vehicle for a few minutes, breathing slowly and deeply, calming myself before sitting with her. We then worked on some simple breathing exercises together before I began. I was able to hear her more clearly as she led me through my work. I was less anxious and more focused.

Mental/Emotional Layer

Our mental state consists of our impressions of information and inputs from the outer world. The input from our senses creates our emotional state. What stories and thoughts have you focused on today? Have you been listening to contentious talk radio or to soothing or uplifting music? Have you been in an argument with someone, or just completed a tough assignment at work? Are you calm and collected from having tea with a friend or going to a meeting or meditating?

As my mental condition could have been influenced by recent activity, I planned time alone before meeting with my sponsor. To avoid arriving rushed, I scheduled our meeting. I also made sure we had open-ended time, so I didn't have to cut the visit short. If you haven't been sharing along the way as you worked our Fourth Step, sitting down to go over the Fifth Step may take a long time, perhaps many hours. If this is the case, you may want to schedule a few meetings so you don't become depleted on any level of your koshas. Plus, you don't want to exhaust your sponsor.

Wisdom Layer

Our intellectual and discerning layer may be challenged in Step Five. We use the discerning mind to evaluate actions and intentions according to higher values and beliefs. This appraisal may have drained us. Using the yamas, niyamas, and other principles to examine and reevaluate our life is hard work. Going over it again as we share will be tiring, too. So, keep in mind that reaffirming your ethics and your spiritual beliefs helps to strengthen them. Prepare yourself to share deeply from your heart and mind. My sponsor had me sit quietly beside her. When it was needed, we would again take several breaths together. Occasionally, she would stop me and ask what I believed now. She would ask what greater good I could find in myself now. She repeatedly brought my attention back to the powerful new moral choices I was currently making, as evidence of my growth and improved judgment.

Spiritual/Bliss Layer

Take a few moments to celebrate your heart, your compassion, and your joy. Sharing our story in Step Five is hard—only because we care more, know better, and believe differently than we did before. If we hadn't changed, if we did not have a stronger sense of right and wrong or of who we are, then this process and information wouldn't bother us.

Before you meet with your sponsor, take some breaths of gratitude and appreciation for yourself: you have come so far. It is a painful process because you are good, and you care. Service to others—opening your heart to the divine spirit in us all, to your higher power, and to the divinity within yourself—will give you the courage to speak honestly when you meet with your sponsor.

Chakras and Step Five

Take a few moments to check in with your chakras in Step Five.

Root Chakra

How grounded do you feel? If you feel impulsive or reckless, need approval, or are overly cautious, then your root chakra might be overactive or underactive. Walking in a park, being close to nature, and breathing deeply into the belly can balance this chakra. Take some time for yourself in order to feel stable.

Sacral Chakra

Do you feel overly proud after completing Step Four, or do you feel emotionally blocked and introverted? Your sacral chakra may be too active or blocked. Doing something creative can clear it. Movement and yoga can help the energy flow. Finding comfort and feeling good about ourselves may seem elusive at this time, but finding a way to approach feelings of joy can help.

You have done good work: you have taken the time to look inward and evaluate things you have done and said, and you have an idea that you don't want to repeat the useless or damaging things. You may have discovered some forgotten goodness as well. Remember these. This is a reason to celebrate your work up to this point. Meditation, massage, or a meeting can help bring this chakra into balance.

Solar Plexus Chakra

Feeling judgmental or isolated is among the emotions that can indicate an overactive or blocked solar plexus chakra. Our sense of self-esteem resides here. Feeling too proud or too insignificant will not help us as we work the steps. There is wisdom to be found in the solar plexus chakra, which is the location of our gut-brain, or belly-brain—a part of our physiology that holds and transmits emotions. This complex part of our anatomy is independent of the thinking brain and the central nervous system.

Before you go to see your sponsor to spill your guts, it is wise to check in with yourself and find balance. Self-acceptance is a key to finding and right-sizing ourselves. Gratitude and acceptance can lead to a grounded sense of contentment that can ease a barbed-wire stomach, alleviating gut-wrenching anxiety or fear.

Read some affirmations, speak kindly to yourself, reaffirm that you have done a good and complete job in your Step Four, and be easy on yourself. I have several books of affirmations, and opening one at random frequently gives me the message that I need to reframe my worldview and speak more kindly to myself.

Heart Chakra

If you become jealous or worried about others' achievements or work on their steps, your heart chakra may be overactive. If you are lacking in self-worth or self-compassion, you may need to reenergize your heart chakra. Step Four is heavy, and sharing it with my sponsor did encourage me to take an honest look at the wreckage of my past. I was disappointed in myself, a little angry, and ashamed. These feelings were valid, but they weren't the whole story: I was also brave, ready to change, and doing the best I could at any given time. However, I was also not doing as well as I hoped.

I sabotaged my sense of worth when I was prepared to meet with my sponsor the first time through. I compared my Fourth Step to the stories I had heard in meetings. I remember only those who spoke about the length, the depth, and the all-encompassing investigation they had done. I was afraid I hadn't been as thorough as they had. I second-guessed myself numerous times. I wasn't sure I was ready to share because I wasn't sure it was perfect—yet.

I later came to know that doubt was part of the process, and I noted the feelings and moved through them. I was going to doubt myself, be unsure, and then take steps to reassure myself and proceed to my sponsor's house.

To balance the heart chakra, find companionship and care. Find it with others and find it within yourself. Speak kindly to yourself, using friendly words and phrases. If you are familiar with *metta* meditation, spend some time in loving kindness meditation to strengthen your resolve. Rather than moving in haste, take your time to prepare your heart for this soulful sharing.

Throat Chakra

What could be more honest than telling your story to another person in a safe space? This story is not to be told to just anyone and everyone. It is between you and a trusted friend, a person who will treat your words with confidence and respect. Ensuring that the throat chakra is flowing freely will help us tremendously as we tell our truth. If we are stubbornly resisting the Fifth Step, or if we are feeling hyperactive or rushing into it, we may need to work on our throat chakra.

Drinking water or lukewarm tea, singing, or chanting aloud can bring you back in touch with your throat chakra in a harmonious way.

Third Eye Chakra

A key to unlocking our new dreams and goals is the third eye chakra. Letting the energy flow through the third-eye chakra gives us wisdom and insight as we share our inventory. If we are blocked, we may experience self-doubt or become fearful or worrisome. If the energy here is running out of control, we may be impatient or oversensitive.

Finding clear movement and equilibrium in the third eye chakra will help you sit with your feelings as you share with your sponsor. I rushed into my first iteration of my Fourth Step. I was totally out of balance, and both my work and my sharing reflected this. Later, I saw this sharing as a doorway to my new self. I saw and heard my own values in Step Five, their shadow side in Step Four, and their bright side in my hopes for the future.

To free the energy of the third eye chakra, I practiced reading and repeating positive affirmations. Lighting incense or candles scented with sandalwood, clary sage, or rosemary can also stimulate and balance this chakra.

Crown Chakra

Isolation, disconnection, and feeling not just unique but profoundly different from others can be signs of a blocked crown chakra. When these sensations and perceptions occur, our crown chakra is out of balance and can be particularly challenging. Through the Fifth Step, we reconnect to the group and ourselves—not only by the story we tell but also by having told it. If we shortchange ourselves by avoiding this work, we may deny ourselves the experience of reconnection.

I cannot tell you how many times I rescheduled a meeting with my sponsor at this point in working the steps. This most recent time through the steps, however, we were able to discuss my pattern and address it. I created a strategy for myself to avoid repeating this charade. I set an intention to arrange an appointment I could make and then meet it, no matter what. It was liberating to break the cycle of avoidance. I did so by practicing discipline and self-care evaluations and strategies, which I did by looking at the koshas and my energy centers. I realized I would feel uncomfortable, but I didn't need to run.

Gunas and Step Five

Using the quality of movement in rajas and forgoing the draw of the dark, sedentary attribute of tamas, I started to effect change. The first time I anticipated doing Step Five with my sponsor, I felt flushed and tired. That became my excuse to reschedule my meeting with her. On another occasion, feelings of depression and fearfulness dragged me down. I experienced a lethargy that was emotionally and physically draining. In cycling between rajas and tamas, I realized that heavy listlessness had been preceded by a period of frenetic activity. I was done with my Fourth Step, and I couldn't wait to go to a meeting and let everyone know I had finished it. I was unfocused at my job and jumpy with the kids for a few days. Then the darkness descended, and I wanted to avoid the thought of the Fourth and Fifth Steps. My feeling of joy was dampened by the fear of sharing it with my higher power and sponsor.

I teeter-tottered between overexcitement and lassitude for two or three days during my initial time through Step Five. The next time, the swing was a little less extreme, and I have come to recognize the cycle. I know I need to rest, but not to withdraw. I need the movement of rajas to make the change, but the intent of the mobility is not only for the sake of motion but also to move toward harmony.

Putting It All Together

Above all, taking the time to check in and see how we feel, to sense the state of our balance on any and all levels of the chakras and the koshas, can greatly assist in our preparation to discuss our fourth-step inventory. I was lucky in that I was able to sit with my sponsor and put some of these self-care practices into action. Kindness and self-care lay the groundwork for wise speech and wise listening.

The challenge in this work is to look beyond the drama to find the dharma. Over the years, all my sponsors helped me with this. Sharing the results of our Fourth Step requires trust and finding a compassionate listener. Listen and watch your sponsor. You will see unconditional love. Experience this toward yourself. This is the beginning of grounding and trusting in yourself. You can now grow in a wholesome direction.

This is the time to practice restorative yoga, a practice of supported poses, held for long periods of time. This is a way to treat yourself with tenderness as you allow another person to guide you in a soothing, self-healing practice. Wear cool, comfy clothes to class and bring a lavender-scented eye pillow if the studio doesn't have one for you to borrow. Use more support than you think you need, move more slowly than you thought possible, and stay in the calmness of the present moment. As you evaluate what is going on, you can practice the choice of finding alternative, positive attitudes and support.

Pose for Step Five: Supported Sphinx Pose

You may want to use stacked towels or your bolster for this pose. The supported sphinx pose strengthens the back as well as giving it flexibility; doing Step Five requires strength as well as resilience. In this pose, you are prone but gazing forward. The upraised heart offers openness, allowing for strength and courage. You care for yourself at the same time you open up.

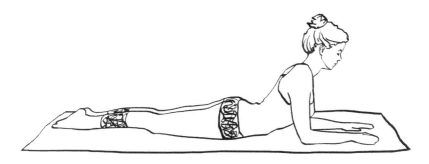

To Come Into the Pose

Lie on your belly facing the ground. In the unsupported pose, bring your elbows to the ground under your shoulders with your forearms on the ground, parallel to one another and in front of you. Using the strength of your arms, keep your chest lifted off the ground, being sure to keep the hip bones firmly planted on the mat. Your legs actively extend behind you. Your gluteus muscles draw back toward the heels. Simple yet complicated, this is a powerful pose. To add another dimension to the pose, you can put towels or a softer bolster between your chest and the floor. Try different things that will allow you to stay in this position for two to five minutes. Tolerating healthy discomfort is part of the process of opening up to another person.

To Get Out of the Pose

Retract your hand to beneath your shoulders. Then, rock back on your heels into child's pose. Using the same props, supports, or other comfortable arrangement, stay here for at least one minute as you return to sanity. Have your notebook ready so you can write down your thoughts about the pose, the process, and your feelings.

"When disturbed with negative thoughts,
cultivate positive thoughts."

SUTRA 2.33

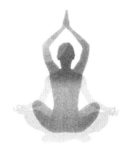

Chapter Six

FINDING WHAT WORKS

—— STEP SIX ——

We were entirely ready to have God remove
all these defects of character.

Step Six is the first of two steps that receive only the briefest mention in the Big Book—one paragraph each. They are investigated in more thorough fashion in the *Twelve and Twelve*. Some non-traditional literature evaluates them together; however, they will be treated as two distinct steps here. Steps Six and Seven are deep steps that can provide a lifelong journey for self-improvement. If negative self-talk and a judging internal dialogue are habits, these, too, can be addressed in practicing Step Six.

Willingness is the core of Step Six. To become ready is to become willing, and this involves the intention to improve. There are a variety of approaches to ameliorating defensive and destructive behaviors that impair willingness. We can employ strategies to grant us security and serenity. Once grounded and composed, we can imagine letting go of some of our less desirable aspects of character. We can't stay the same and change, too. To change requires action, and there are a few ways to take action in Step Six.

One fellowship suggests listing our defects of character on slips of paper and sorting them into three piles: those we are ready to give up, those we can't yet give up, and those we believe we will never be ready to give up. As we go through our day, we should take notice of all these characteristics and consider how they serve us.

In a Step Six workshop of another fellowship, it is suggested that we look into the ability to be willing and the ability to let go of the burden of doing things alone, without our spiritual guide and higher power. We should list the defects and see under what circumstances we *could* let them go. This guidance is specific in recommending that we start off with "resentments, jealousy, pride, and procrastination." As in other recovery groups, it is suggested that we examine how each of these defects keeps us where we are, impeding our growth.

My first experience with Step Six was to read the Big Book and say, "Yay! I am ready to be perfect! Who wouldn't be? Take it all!!!" Then I went on to read Step Seven, after which I used one of my defects—perfectionism—to package the rest of my deficiencies in a bundle. I then sat back and waited to be struck wonderful. How ironic it was that this should be my attitude, when the title of the Big Book chapter that includes this step is "Into Action." It was not called "Into Waiting." Luckily, I stuck around long enough to realize there really was something to *do* here.

As yoga is not a religious practice—nor is recovery—I look at the word *God* as shorthand for higher power. When I am working with women, I offer this concept to them. Some are comfortable with the word *God,* while others are put off by it. That can become a stumbling block—sometimes a boulder on which to crash and burn. The semantics become the focus of the step rather than the powerful message that it is time to get ready for a powerful change to take place. Our higher power, our spiritual support, or our internal compass awaits our permission to guide us through the profound changes necessary to create a new life.

Are you ready? Will you let your higher power guide your authentic self to light? Will you allow a steadfast voice for positive change guide you away from the hell you have created for yourself? This has been the attitude or the point of view I have offered the women I sponsor. Avoid getting hung up on the word *God* and look for meaning. Allow the invitation of Step Six to manifest in your life.

Step Four can be a living document of recovery. With my sponsor, I could both whittle down the exaggerations and evaluate what really were complaints or excuses for my behaviors. This ultimately led to a list of attributes and behaviors that I repeated over and over—my sixth-step defects. These were conventional ways I reacted when insecure, afraid, or angry, or when experiencing some other form of vulnerability. They were attitudes I had held when resentful, jealous, or comparing myself to others. I had patterns of behavior when feeling needy or wanting attention. There were unattractive ways I acted when hungry, angry, lonely, or tired. Every form of illusion, delusion, false understanding, or disconnection from my fellows was to be found among my defenses and defects of character. Step Six offered the opportunity to revisit those character defects I had honed in my active addiction.

I became willing to let go of them all. The fear that impeded my ability to totally unclench my fist surrounding these characteristics was that of the unknown. If I didn't do these things, how would I be protected? How would I feel safe, cared for, or secure? How would I remain in charge? How would I forecast and prepare for the way things would unfold? Those were the great questions, and they were the unacknowledged quicksand beneath my desire to change.

To become ready for the defects to be removed, I needed to create some emotional and spiritual scaffolding to keep me secure. My intention to "grow along spiritual lines" was of great importance. Before I embarked on my journey into yoga, the desire to practice a loving life had been present in my subconscious. As a child, I wanted to be loving and kind, get along with others, do my part, play fairly, and do all of those other things we learned in kindergarten.

These childhood lessons were valuable, but life became complicated with family chaos. I adapted by developing character defects and defenses. Later, I contributed chaos of my own, creating more bad habits and incorrect behaviors. I needed to go back to the basics of a loving life, and I needed to do so in emotional safety. Yoga has helped me unravel the insidious nature of my defects and given me tools to protect and ground myself while I do so.

Yamas and Step Six

Practicing the restraints, or yamas, will help us avoid continuing down the path of harmful, destructive behavior. Finding out what is holding us back from practicing non-harming, non-lying, non-stealing, non-excess, and non-attachment can alert us when we need to focus on these virtues. As we let go of defensive behaviors, it is important for us to know and believe the following statement, so we can be grounded and stable: I am not a bad person trying to become a good one; I am a good person getting ready to let go of incorrect conduct.

I wondered what I had put in the place of the restraints. Digging a little deeper into motivations and using yogic tools, I was able to investigate my impressions and my sensory and emotional inputs, find my balance, and explore my interior goodness. On the mat, I was able to connect with my body, my breath, and my spirit in a compassionate way. I continue to use the yamas in relation to myself and others.

Niyamas and Step Six

Another way to gain a foundation in healing and self-care is to practice the niyamas, particularly contentment and surrender. With gratitude and acceptance, we can see ourselves as we are. This can foster contentment, and I discovered this was a place to start. Rather than jumping ahead to the image of the perfect person I wanted to be, I learned to accept myself as I was: a person working toward better behavior inside and out. Surrender would become more important in Step Seven, but being ready to have my defects removed was the preparation for this release and became part of my vocabulary.

Asana and Step Six

The yoga mat is a wonderful place to physically establish where we are in this moment. A fluctuating mind will make balance poses challenging. I have learned that trying to be in an extended pose beyond what my ability and flexibility authentically allow will bring discomfort and cause me to lose the precision of proper alignment, possibly harming me. This reminds me to acknowledge my present self.

Reaching beyond where I am in this exact moment, literally and figuratively, does me no good. Scrupulous attention to how I can be in the pose and move from pose to pose with authenticity will prepare me for a new pose, a new day, and a new challenge taken in safety. I sample each pose and work within it to find the point of effort. As we say at the end of each fellowship meeting, "It works if you work it, and you're worth it." In my physical practice, I get immediate feedback when I find the balance of neither overworking nor undertrying.

Practicing the poses can also help us find grounding. When we are grounded, have practiced breathing and moving, and are rested, we are more able to consider change. Step Six is about embracing change—a change to something we do not yet know. It is not change from one job or home to another; it is change from doing, or not doing, to action, or inaction, and moving on to something we have previously not tried or experienced before. This is a true unknown.

Using the same process as used in asana—curiosity without judgment—take a look at how you exhibit feelings of anger, resentment, or procrastination. How could appreciation of others be enhanced by avoiding jealousy or covetousness? The agitation of dissatisfaction might go away. How would your energy and clarity of thought improve? Referring back to the list you created with the help of your sponsor, continue on through the list of characteristics. When contemplating change, it is best if we are rested and grounded. A hatha yoga practice can give us that.

Kleshas and Step Six

The kleshas are ripe for examination in Step Six. How do you invoke them to avoid readiness? How do false thinking, ego, craving, and aversion shake up your stability and guard your old traits?

I have a mental image of my addiction as a creature that wants me back under its complete control. It weakens me by making me feel separate and isolated. When I feel alone and fearful, I am more likely to revert to an old way of thinking, and possibly to an old way of behaving, such as drinking, using, sexual indiscretion, or compulsive eating or shopping. The obstacles, including fear, separate me from myself, others, and my higher power. They rock my world, and not in a good way.

Meditation and Step Six

Meditation, which is suggested in Step Eleven, can be part of our life at any time. It is one of the practices of yoga often included as part of a regular class or on its own in a special workshop. Trying several styles and types of meditation can help us find one that works. What meditation can offer as part of the readiness portion of Step Six is another way to get grounded—to let go of the "what ifs" in relation to releasing our character defects. It is the ultimate practice of letting go.

Whether listening to a guided meditation or practicing in silence, I continue to release my attachment to my thoughts. They, like bad habits, recur spontaneously, and I practice letting them go. Even though the thoughts return, I have more and more experience in releasing them. I have developed a different relationship with my thoughts. They are not facts—they are not real. I let them drift as I gain more skill in non-attachment.

Chakras and Step Six

Balancing the root, sacral, and solar plexus chakras is key to feeling connected, grounded, and comfortable in our skin. Security, integration, intimacy, and self-confidence are signs of balanced chakras. Each of our character defects can result from, or be exacerbated by, a chakra being out of balance.

Referring to my Fourth Step, and to the memories of what had gone on in my life, I discovered I had a lot of pent-up emotions. I bottled them up, so my energies were blocked. When feelings came out, it was to an inappropriate degree. They were often expressed toward someone who was not party to the stifled issues and/or about a totally unrelated topic. For example, I had been harboring feelings of being unappreciated for years. Later, I would burst out with venom at my friend for ignoring me when she appeared to be preoccupied around me—years of pent-up anger rolled out and onto her. My reaction was out of proportion with the event. The bottled-up energy of anger burst forth.

This event that I mention showed up in my Fourth Step, which allowed me to look at anger in my Sixth Step. The history was that the energy of holding onto anger—which may have been fitting for situations in my youth—turned into rage by the time it was expressed. Feeling grounded in my root chakra now allows me to express anger in a proper degree and at the proper time by letting go of the well of anger and being ready for the next phase of healing.

I also wanted to be ready to change my attitude about how I manifested my sexuality. I had a history of unhealthy sexual experiences, I had experienced sexual trauma, and I had treated myself poorly, like a commodity. I worked through the events and the underlying issues with my sponsor in my Fifth Step in addition to seeking outside professional help. In Step Six, I wanted to be ready to look at myself and my relationships differently. The sacral chakra is the seat of sexual energy. I didn't know how my defects and my erroneous attitude about sex and intimacy would play out. I had no idea what a healthy relationship was.

I didn't know how to act in, communicate in, or navigate a relationship when sexuality was not something to be bartered. I longed to be cherished and regarded for my character, for myself, but I didn't have faith or trust that I would be enough. In connecting with my sacral chakra and finding balance there, I prepared myself for the unknown—a new, healthy way to regard myself and others. In working on this and finding health in my sexuality, I have been able to have a loving, intimate relationship for many years.

As the child of an alcoholic, I was used to living in a home of chaos. I knew my parents loved me, but that love showed itself in conflicting ways. One moment they told me I could be anything I wanted to be; the next moment they told me I could do nothing right. I was wonderful one minute and a fatso the next. I was also a child with the responsibilities of an adult. The inside didn't match the outside, and the outside was always changing. Was I ready to improve my confidence and self-esteem? Absolutely! But did I deserve it? I was unsure. In balancing the solar plexus chakra, I have made a step toward embracing my true self with confidence—a truly foreign feeling but one critical to becoming truly integrated.

Koshas and Step Six

When we use the koshas to evaluate how we feel, checking our readiness to change at all levels, we might discover that they are not in sync. We need to take some time to evaluate ourselves thoroughly—physically, energetically, emotionally, intellectually, joyfully, and spiritually.

When I do this, I might find that my energetic and physical bodies are ready to make changes, for I am rested, I am fed, and I am prepared to take Step Six. However, my intellectual/emotional kosha isn't so sure. It is tender and vulnerable, and it questions what life will be like if I do things another way.

My wisdom kosha, which can be more judging than discerning when not in a state of harmony, may be critical rather than supportive. When disconnection occurs, I lose contact with my higher power, which is detrimental to my well-being and enthusiasm for change. Reestablishing the connection with my guiding spirit is one way I reintegrate. Sitting with my feelings and letting them flow without comment or criticism can bring the observing mind back to being a witness and away from being a judge.

A lot of restructured self-talk goes on in this process of preparing for Step Six. As we get ready for change, the fundamental words we use when talking to ourselves change and soften to allow the transition to occur.

Putting It All Together

In getting ready to have my defects removed, I have used a compassionate language of self-talk and a positive voice to help and reassure me. I have even become ready for the internal dialogue to change. The discussion in our heads, the "committee" we hear about in the rooms, needs to prepare for change. When you are balanced, secure, and connected to your higher power, you are entirely ready to move toward your enlightened inner being.

Pose for Step Six: Crocodile Pose

Release into the floor with this pose. Let the ground hold you up while you focus on your breathing, the sensations of filling and emptying the body. Preparing to have defects of character removed can be both freeing and overwhelming. Remain aware of all seven chakras from below the navel up to the crown of the head while you lie there. What are you experiencing at each position? This is a time to reflect as you lie there and breathe.

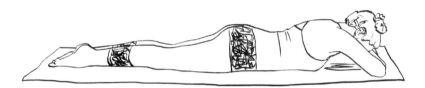

To Come Into the Pose

This is a simple belly-lying position with your arms crossed at the top of the mat above your head and your head resting either with forehead down or with a cheek on stacked hands. Have your ankles hip width apart and have your feet flop whichever way they are most comfortable. Pay attention to releasing into the floor as thoroughly as you can. Breathe. Stay here for five to seven minutes. If you have chosen to put a cheek on your stacked hands, turn your head in the other direction halfway through the pose. Your mind may wander. If it does, ask it to come back to consciousness of the body, the chakras, and the desire to let go of ways of being that no longer serve you.

To Get Out of the Pose

When you are done, bring your hands under your shoulders, push down, and fold back into child's pose. Rest for a few breaths, then sit up on your heels, swivel around, and sit with your legs extended out for a few moments before moving on.

This has been a well-deserved rest after working on the step. Write down in your notebook any revelations you have about yourself, any reservations you have about the process, and what your attitude may be as you move on from Step Six.

"These afflictions can be subdued, as the causes
of suffering were, by tracing them back to
their origin or through meditation."

SUTRA 4.28

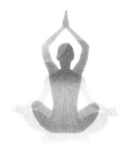

Chapter Seven

LETTING GO OF WHAT NO LONGER WORKS

— STEP SEVEN —

We humbly asked Him to remove our shortcomings.

In Steps Four through Six, I investigated how I had behaved in my active addiction. I also looked at some of the reasons why, but I didn't investigate the actions of others, find an excuse, or create a list of excuses, such as "I stole from her because she shorted me on my drugs" or "I resented my parents because they didn't treat me fairly." The root of the "whys" was traced to underlying feelings of scarcity, low self-worth, or need. Anger and fear can cause unpleasant or regrettable actions. The basis for them may have been insecurity or unmet needs. The fundamental or original issues underlying those negative behaviors could have been discovered in the Fourth and Fifth Steps.

For example, I discovered that my anxiety and insecurity overrode the values I had as a child. My perfectionism caused me to be hypercritical of others and myself. This, coupled with the selfishness common to those suffering from the disease of addiction, caused me to be careless in my actions. These traits were rooted in my desire to be accepted and to avoid disappointing others, fearing my mistakes could lead to rejection. My resentments kept me from getting close to others. Healthy intimacy was too risky; I hadn't been able to trust anyone.

In Step Seven, I came to terms with these shortcomings. With my sponsor, I listed the characteristics that had often been major drivers in my life. During this step, I was simply, without fanfare, without anticipating a specific result, asking that they be removed.

The seventh-step prayer from the Big Book and other recovery literature is used to embrace what we ask for at this time:

> My Creator, I am now willing that you should have all
> of me, good and bad. I pray that you now remove from
> me every single defect of character which stands in the
> way of my usefulness to you and my fellows. Grant me
> strength, as I go out from here, to do your bidding.

This prayer of appeal embraces not only acceptance but also the dark and the light of our being. It asks that whatever is needed be available. It expresses the desire to be useful to those we come in contact with and the hope that we retain our courage as we do this.

As a yogini, I break this prayer down into pieces and apply it to my understanding, as I believe in my version of a higher power. This can be referred to as "taking what [I] can use and leaving the rest."

There is a specific plea that we do God's bidding or command. This is where that authentic relationship with a higher power is of great importance. Employing the word *God* or any other name or phrase is not as important as the understanding behind the word as a spiritual guide to our growth and change. We want to be a contributing member of our society. Let whatever characteristics we have be present to the degree needed to have us be able to do what is needed in the world.

In the first three steps, we developed a relationship with a higher power. If this has floundered from then to now, then we can't take Step

Seven yet. At a meeting, I heard that if you have problems with a step, then you need to back up to the step before it. From time to time, I have had to back up through several steps, refreshing my understanding of my higher power and my commitment before moving ahead. It was the honest thing to do. I needed to refresh my concept of a higher power and revitalize and reaffirm that relationship. Once I did that, I could go on authentically to Step Seven.

Rather than taking the literal meaning from the last line of the Seventh Step Prayer, I like to replace it with the following text, which I paraphrased from a fellow yogi: "Let me be where I need to be, doing what I need to be doing with the people I need to meet. I would like my shortcomings to be removed to the extent that is necessary for me to be helpful and useful in my life. That is all." When I strive for perfection, I do so out of ego and become self-serving. That is not the intent of Step Seven. We are humble, simple, and true to ourselves. This is not a self-aggrandizing step.

At a recent meeting, I heard a person speak about Step Seven. It was eye-opening because I hadn't internalized the wisdom in this way before. What I remember being said was, "When I modestly ask for my shortcomings to be removed, I have asked that they challenge me so I could experience how I would act and respond were they fully removed. How will I know if my impatience is being removed unless I have situations that make me impatient? If I want to become less quick to anger, I may have to endure some antagonistic events to experience calm."

After that comment was made, I understood that during Step Seven I need to include circumstances such as when I want to be more compassionate with myself and my awareness of less acceptable attributes may increase. This is how I will know that I am moving toward releasing what no longer works. I have let my higher power, my universal spirit, the goodness and wisdom of my inner self, allow me to respond in a different way than from my shortcomings. Yoga has helped me to see what was no longer working and has guided me on how to act according to my ethics and my values, repurposing myself to become truer to my being.

How do we get humble? The word *humble* gets a lot of attention at meetings. Many are concerned that finding humility is similar to being humiliated. Once again, we may become embroiled in the semantics and lose the meaning. Choosing a definition that means "respectful"—an admirable quality that does not involve putting oneself above another—can ameliorate this concern. In asking our higher power to remove our shortcomings, we leave the heavy lifting to our higher power and abstain from taking the lead. We lay all the issues out and then see what happens. We don't choose. That would not be humble.

On the other hand, we need to take action and behave differently. When in alignment with our spiritual self, we make different choices than we had made while in our active addiction, or when we were self-centered. We have been moving away from the self-serving motives of active addiction and early recovery. That is our footwork. What comes out of that decision is up to our higher power.

Action is necessary; change is required. In recovery we say, "If you keep doing what you've always done, you will keep getting what you've always gotten." A recovery-oriented comedian, Mark Lundholm, has the tagline, "First Thought Wrong." That is funny because in early recovery that is often true. Later on in recovery, it may be wiser to encourage a more positive internal dialogue and begin to foster healthy first thoughts.

Developing a new mind habit is a way to release shortcomings. Practicing second thoughts can help them become *first* thoughts, which makes the initial thought the right idea. Rather than coming from a place of self-doubt, we can move toward self-trust. We can create new habits of thinking.

Samskara and Step Seven

If we are critical in our head, we will be more critical of others. If we are short-tempered in our internal conversations, we will exhibit short-tempered traits. When anxious, we exude anxiety. Any one of our shortcomings will be expressed according to our mind's habits. These habits have been developed over years of protecting ourselves, navigating an unfriendly world, and trying to make sense of chaos.

With very few guideposts or leaders, I was trying to maneuver through a life I didn't understand. I heard negative messages about myself and the world. I lived in places where my gender and my race were disparaged. These experiences influenced me and how I saw the world. They influenced how I viewed myself *in* the world and others around me.

In the first six steps, I opened my eyes to the effects these habits had on myself and on others. In Step Seven, I surrendered them without hesitation. With aware intention about my actions, my behaviors, and my mental outlook, I developed new, positive samskara.

Karma and Step Seven

The yogic ideal of natural consequences is karma, which is complex. In its original context, the sages meant that karma could flow down from our ancestors. In another context, we could discuss the generational impact of addiction and other family system disorders and how they affect subsequent generations, definable as an effect of generational karma.

I am not discussing karma as it moves through the generations of a family here. Karma is not an immediate result of an action; it comes when it comes. We sometimes use the word *karma* in place of the old-fashioned word *comeuppance,* meaning a negative outcome as the result of thoughtless action. There are qualities of karma as well. Harmful action with harmful intent is different from harmful action out of ignorance or inattention. Positive, helpful action performed out of ego, or the desire to be thanked, is better than an accidental bad action, but it is not as pure as a positive action taken without thought of acknowledgment or reward. There is all manner of shading in between and among those four types, and there is no external judge of the actions. It is all based on intention and leaving the result to our higher power.

In applying karma to Step Seven, we make an intention to take right action and then let go. We hope that our shortcomings will be relieved so that the best result can manifest. We will find out if the shortcomings have been altered entirely, or if we merely experience a sustained removal for a length of time. In my case, most shortcomings have been ameliorated but not removed completely. It all depends on my spiritual condition.

Kleshas and Step Seven

Yoga differentiates between the seer self—the internal, eternal self—and the part of the self that records or interprets what is felt, experienced, touched, or seen. Our external experience of being—such as gender identification, race, socioeconomic experience, age, and education—may be mistakenly called our real self. However, this outer, external being is always changing, so it isn't the true self; it is merely the current experience of the self.

This is a complicated idea, and it took me a while to appreciate it. I realized that I had been holding onto certain characteristics as they created a role for me. I was the kid of an alcoholic, so I became resentful of my parents. I unintentionally acted in a certain way as a result of this identity. In my active addiction, I was a free-love person with no boundaries around my sexuality. This resulted in harms and broken relationships due to my false identification with this concept. I was a good worker, so I went to my job, even when I was incompetent due to a hangover or a lingering intoxication. Consequently, I cheated my employers out of adequate service. My bad decisions arose from my identification with a role rather than out of my seer self, my atman. This true self was nowhere to be found when I was using, and even in early recovery my true self could not be expressed until I worked through the steps.

When we get stuck in an identity, we experience the obstacle of ego: attachment. If we hold onto our identity as one who holds a grudge, is intolerant, and has too much to do to be patient with others, we are holding onto a role. By not abiding to our true inner self, we are blocking the removal of our shortcomings. In humility, or letting go of control and releasing a false front, we can finally have these shortcomings—our defenses—removed.

Yamas, Niyamas, and Step Seven

Non-excess, non-attachment, cleanliness, and surrender are yamas and niyamas that can assist in Step Seven. Letting go of excess, seeking moderation (chastity), cleanliness of action and spirit, and surrender to one's higher power are all part of humility and asking for help. When we are our right size—neither knowing better nor being better nor being obsequious or insignificant—we are ready. When ready, we are willing; when willing, we can authentically ask our higher power for help. Even while having our shortcomings removed, we need to practice patience, avoid self-criticism, and learn to trust.

Chakras and Step Seven

Connecting with your crown chakra can be very useful in Step Seven, for it is our source of enlightenment and spiritual connection. Using the image of the lotus flower emerging from the mud, I imagine my recovering self as I rise from the muck of my past. Connection to our higher power releases us from the confines of our physical body and our ego, mind, and intellect.

Working toward liberation from the shackles of old behavior, we can open to a brighter, lighter alignment with our true being. We can assist this process by practicing affirmations or receiving inspiration from nature, art, and serene sounds. We can balance our crown chakra with visualizations, prayer, and meditation. Step Seven begins the gifts we will give to ourselves and others in our recovery.

Putting It All Together

The phrase "in God's time, not mine" comes to mind when I think of Step Seven. We remain at the ready, and, little by little, we can see changes. I had at first expected I would be struck wonderful when I read Step Six and had said yes to Step Seven. Yet, after working Step Six and coming to Step Seven, I realized the change would be gradual and I would need to reaffirm my dedication repeatedly. With patience as to timing and manner of these profound changes, you will be amazed by the changes. These happen moment by moment, but you will only recognize them after years in recovery.

Pose for Step Seven: Reclined Twist

Use a bolster for support and a towel or blanket for a headrest. Twists are said to detoxify—and isn't that what we want to do when humbly asking that our shortcomings be removed? We want to be detoxified of those attributes that no longer serve others or us.

You have prepared yourself in the other steps and poses. You are now ready to ask to be relieved of the excesses that have manifested themselves into negative, unhelpful behavior patterns. You do this while asking for support, though; you don't rely on doing it yourself. You allow for help. Move in the direction of the twist and then release into the power of the twist.

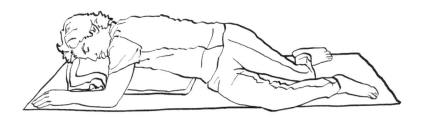

To Come Into the Pose

Set the bolster on the mat, which has been placed at least a foot from a wall or piece of furniture. Place the bolster lengthwise in the center of the mat and put the folded towel or blanket across the top fifth or so of the bolster. Place your right hip below and against the bottom of the bolster, and tuck your folded legs behind you. Move your torso to face the bolster, placing one hand on either side of the bolster. Keep turning until you reach your comfortable limit, then lie down on the bolster.

You can turn your head to face away from your bent knees if your neck is comfortable with that amount of twist. If not, just place your forehead on the pillow made by your towel or blanket, or turn your head and place it down facing the in same direction as your knees. Try all the variations and choose the most sustainable.

Release exertion in your arms as soon as your head and neck are comfortable. Let the ground and your props hold you up. Breathe deeply here for no more than five minutes.

Before switching to your other side, follow the directions for getting out of the pose. Then repeat, starting with the left hip at the edge of the bolster. Twist to face the bolster and find comfort on this side. It should be a balance between effort in the twist and ease in finding support.

To Get Out of the Pose

Put your palms on the floor at either side of the bolster. Push down as you raise your torso. Turn your back toward the bolster. Extend your legs and pause for five long, deep breath cycles. Breathe in and out with attention.

Use your notebook to record your physical response to the twist. This is a powerful pose, and some moments of reflection can be useful. Make notes about your response to the work on Step Seven. Can you turn your shortcomings over freely now?

"Once the mind is freed of the veils of misperceptions and concealing truths, there is little left to be revealed."

SUTRA 4.31

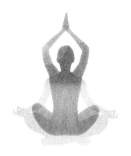

Chapter Eight
CONSIDERING CONSEQUENCES

— STEP EIGHT —

We made a list of all persons we had harmed,
and became willing to make amends to them all.

Step Eight is the step of brotherly love, of compassion, and for truly considering the consequences of our past choices. This step has many places where we can trip: the list, the harms, the willingness, and the making of amends.

Which part do we typically avoid or refute first? I don't know if I am the only one, but resistance is my first instinct as I approach any of the steps. Step Eight seemed particularly worrisome: when I completed it, I would have to do Step Nine! I tell my sponsees, who balk at this point, something my sponsor told me: "Only work the step you are on; don't be concerned with the step that is yet to come."

The first time I worked Step Eight, I was in danger of succumbing to my defects of perfectionism and control. My fear and insecurity had risen in anticipation of the work yet to come in the following step, so

I hesitated. Then, I wanted to get it over with to get to the other side, and I rushed to get the list completed.

Making a list *seemed* like a fairly straightforward task—until I began. Going back to my Fourth Step, I noted names of people. Just names. All of them. I was tempted to eliminate names because of the hurts and harms they had done me, but I was encouraged to list everyone and make changes later. I resisted yet again. I had reservations. The first objections were about those people who had hurt me as a child or who had caused me pain for which there had been no fault on my side—things such as an assault, an abandonment, and robberies. Then there were those people who had passed away. I didn't know whether I should include them, but I did. I included those whom I no longer knew how to reach. Without judgment or decision, I wrote down all the names.

I then had to look at the concept of harming. Whom had I harmed, and how? Some harms were fairly evident: violence, stealing, lying, bad behavior, and sexual misconduct. I had to include things I had done and previously excused as being the natural consequence of resentments, such as petty malice, neglect, or controlling behaviors. I had been harsh with my children and had ignored them in my active addiction. I had fought, both physically and verbally, with family, friends, people I knew, and people I didn't know. I had stolen from people close to me and had lied to everyone I had come into contact with at one time or another. It was a way of life.

The *Twelve and Twelve* suggests that we might look at ways in which our will had conflicted with others' wills. It suggests we focus this investigation on occasions in which our impulses clashed with someone else spiritually, emotionally, physically, or mentally. In other words, we could have harmed people in a number of ways and at many levels of their being.

In my newfound value system, I realized that harms could be either active or inactive in nature. They could occur to others as well as myself. Active ways are more obvious, but inactive and more insidious ways of being harmful can be as painful. Passive ways in which I had harmed people included unresponsiveness and lack of engagement. I had neglected my kids, not out of spite, but because I put off caring for them or forgot. I had withheld time, attention, and affection. I lacked trust in people and acted accordingly. Intimacy was totally foreign to me, although I had been in several "close" relationships. The people whom these attitudes, behaviors, and lack of action had affected went on my list.

To complete the components of Step Eight, I used my discipline to write the list and opened my heart-space of interconnectedness to remain willing. I looked honestly at my past to understand the harms. I also needed patience to avoid getting ahead of myself. Rather than focus on the who, the how, and when I would make apologies and amends, I needed to stay focused and do the Eighth Step first. Yoga helped in this endeavor.

Chakras and Step Eight

I began this step by balancing my energy sources, which gave me the equanimity to embrace the difficulty and pain of working Step Eight. It was hard, it was uncomfortable, and the memories flowed. I started by bringing my attention to my chakras, each in order from root to crown, before putting pen to paper. As with Step Four, I checked for imbalances—overactivity or underactivity—at any of the seven levels.

Root Chakra

Are you feeling impulsive, hyperactive, or reckless? Are you feeling manipulative or possessive? Are you seeking approval? We may be too harsh on ourselves, listing every time we can remember having hurt another's feelings, brushing someone off, or having led someone on. We could be trying to please our sponsor or some imagined perfect eighth-step standard. We need to feel grounded and relatively even in our emotions, remaining balanced and connecting with healthy, solution-oriented friends.

Sacral Chakra

Do you feel emotionally shut down, separate, or isolated? Do you feel arrogant, powerful, or proud? In general, I noticed that my go-to condition for the sacral chakra was underactive, in which I felt shut down, my feelings became remote, and I was disconnected. Doing things such as calling my sponsor, going to a meeting, and talking to others helped me reconnect. If we feel overactive in this chakra, similar activities can help us come back into harmony.

Solar Plexus Chakra

Vital to creating a rational, reasonable approach to Step Eight is the solar plexus chakra. The ego and sense of self are faulty when overenergized or underenergized. If we feel unacknowledged, unappreciated, or unable to learn and grow, or if we are judgmental, critical, or stubborn, we are not in the correct space to do Step Eight. We cannot create a proper list when we are like this. We can neither evaluate what harms we have done nor remain willing. Reading affirmations, being in nature, and eating healthy foods, including spices such as turmeric and ginger, can help us balance the solar plexus chakra.

Heart Chakra

In meetings, we learn to kindle and nurture our empathetic abilities. We do this as we listen to one another and work with newcomers. We can hear our feelings expressed by others as they share, learning more about ourselves in the process. We listen to the kind words from our sponsor as he or she encourages us. We also find ourselves reassuring and supporting others with all our heart.

When our heart chakra is balanced and clear, loving energy comes easily, naturally, to us. When this chakra is blocked, we lack compassion, love, and a sense of self-worth. If it is overactive, we feel jealousy, are miserly with our affection, and respond to others as if we were taken advantage of. None of these feelings, mental states, or points of view helps us make our eighth-step list, much less approach it with an authentic desire to make reparations for harms done. We must first take care of the inside in order to go outside. We need to prepare our heart to connect to others in a genuine way.

Practicing acceptance and letting things go can help us heal our heart chakra. Non-attachment is one of the yoga practices involved this process: we use acceptance as part of the practice of cleanliness and the Serenity Prayer as a mantra that can heal the heart.

Throat Chakra

Talking out loud, sharing with our sponsor or at a meeting, or speaking with friends either in person or on the phone is a way to keep the throat chakra in balance. Singing, chanting, and reading affirmations and prayers out loud stimulate this chakra. Rather than relying on internal mind chatter for acknowledgment or approval, or using texts or email correspondence with others, using our own voice is healing. We speak our truth from the throat chakra.

Getting in touch with my truth and my desire to make things right by addressing all the people I had hurt in my addiction started with the list. No better or worse than others—one comes from a centered place of healing awareness. The list itself had to come from an authentic and honest place.

Third Eye Chakra

I prepared myself to consider the consequences of my actions. Often others paid the consequences while I got off relatively scot-free. I drank, used, and ignored or disregarded others. I borrowed a car, and the person loaning it to me had to find it and retrieve it. I found myself in a bad place, physically or emotionally, and someone else had to rescue me. I missed deadlines, and others had to cover for me. I made promises I didn't keep, broke the hearts of people I was involved with, and let down people who trusted me. They paid the price: the poor work, the inconvenience, the hurt, and the disappointment. In more extreme circumstances, they paid for the repairs, covered the rent, and dealt with pain and shame. In my Step Eight, I looked inward to make the honest assessment of who was really harmed, and I added those names to the list.

If the third eye is blocked, we can't see the truth. We lack direction and introspection. Physical and emotional manifestations may include headaches, backaches, depression, or anxiety. To rekindle this chakra, I use my imagination. I see a day when I no longer repeat these behaviors. I use meditation to rekindle the vitality of this important chakra, so I can soften the inward and the outward gaze and bring compassion to the effort of writing my list, realizing my own name needs to be there as well.

Crown Chakra

Yoga poses such as inversions, breath work, and meditation are wonderful for keeping the crown chakra in balance. When it is out of balance and underactive, a feeling of isolation and alienation from others and our higher power can occur. When this chakra is overstimulated, we might become confused or lack empathy. Creating an honest list with an honest desire to address harms done will be more authentic when the crown chakra is in balance.

Addiction is a disease of isolation, and when the chakras are in balance, we experience contented unification with our higher power, with others, and with ourselves. The crown chakra requires our full attention so that genuine freedom and happiness can be found.

Koshas and Step Eight

Using the levels of myself, I made note of how I was feeling. I checked to see if I had a sense of balance and proportion. I examined each layer to see in which way I may have harmed others or myself. I meditated to become centered and calm. I used focused contemplation to deliberate these questions. I first calmed myself with even breath, checked in with my physical and emotional bodies, and determined whether I was falling into a place of overactive, negative self-judgment. Was I able to remain in the role of the observer, merely witnessing my energy, body, and emotions?

Once I settled into the space of the onlooker, I connected with my higher power and let go of directed thoughts. When I felt more grounded, I could pick up my list, check the names, and ask, "How did I negatively affect *them*—energetically, physically, emotionally, mentally, or spiritually?" This was important to know. To get a clearer picture of how I had behaved, I needed to understand the impact of my actions. I looked at my own name and thought about how I had harmed myself using this same paradigm.

Kleshas and Step Eight

There can obstacles that prevent us from proceeding with this step. Two of them may be aversion and our ego.

Aversion

My first Eighth Step was rather brief: I simply listed some names from my Fourth Step without further reflection. Approaching this step from a yogic point of view later in recovery, I looked more deeply into why some names were easy to write down and others were not. With additional reviews of my list, I discovered I was avoiding some names because I was holding onto what they had done to me. I was avoiding others because of shame. I put others down but then erased them because I realized I was not yet willing to make amends to them. I had to back up to willingness and become centered enough to endure the discomfort or pain.

Ego

Whether I was underreporting the names or preparing to apologize too much, my ego was leading me into a false sense of self. As the martyr or the aggressor, I was seeing myself in a single dimension. Disavowing my own feelings or imagining that I had no responsibility for the feelings of others, I was measuring with an erroneous understanding of myself in the world. In yoga, and in my belief about the world, we are universal spirits, each connected to one another. A harm to one is a harm to all. In no case did I not hurt myself when I harmed another. This understanding was another reminder to keep my own name on that list.

Gunas and Step Eight

Moving toward harmony and using the energy of change, I left behind the overwhelming heaviness of tamas. Using the characteristics of rajas, my list began to rocket me toward the fourth dimension of existence, which I would reach through the remaining steps. Before I take action, share a thought, or express myself in any way, including typing or texting, I pause and take stock of where the energy is coming from. Am I moving from sheer excitement without attention to another's feelings? Will I become more balanced and harmonious when all is said and done, or will I remain in a rajasic tumultuous state? Is the energy I am using now frenetic or frantic? When I come from a place of balance, I am in a much more open frame of mind, with more possibilities available than I had previously imagined. I use these considerations when I think about my Eighth Step.

Yamas and Step Eight

Similar to how non-harming, non-lying, non-stealing, non-excess, and non-attachment guided me through the Fourth Step, I used them as I made my list, too. Having the capacity to be honest is a sure guide to helping us complete Step Eight.

Putting It All Together

As I did Step Eight, I had to avoid going overboard. Another inclination of mine was to write down the name of everyone I could remember, whether or not they were mentioned in my Fourth Step. In that effort, I was casting myself as the bad girl, recalling as many circumstances and names as I could. I was overreaching, or being greedy. My false ego was also involved; I wanted it to be lengthy so my list would be sponsor-worthy. In that process, I was hurting myself.

You need to be willing to make amends, but in a way that would also not harm yourself, your self-esteem, and your newfound sense of wholeness. This investigation is not intended as a way for you to punish yourself. It is designed to enable you to find ways you can transform. It signals the beginning of a new life for you, which includes self-care and compassion.

Pose for Step Eight: Supported Fish Pose

Fish pose is a pose that opens your throat and heart. Your head will be connected with the ground close to the crown, so you can connect with internally and externally focused compassion. Your throat will be open and stretched to help you speak the truth. To prepare to speak your truth, you want to tune into your voice, your source of authentic expression. It is also an opportunity to stay connected with your true self. Grab your bolster or fold a pillow lengthwise. Bring a blanket to the mat as well. You will be lying on your back with your head supported.

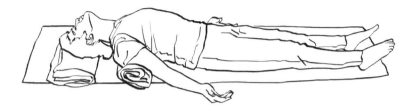

To Come Into the Pose

Place your bolster or folded pillow across your mat about a third of the way down. Put your blanket closer to the top edge. You are going to aim yourself, lying on your back, so that the pillow rests beneath your shoulder blades, your shoulders rest on the mat, and your head tips back onto the blanket.

Sit on the mat with knees bent, soles of the feet on the mat. Place your hands behind your legs and lower yourself easily onto the bolster and the blanket. You may need to adjust your position relative to the props until you get into the position of chest rising and head tipped back. The bolster may be too high, in which case you will need to place a second blanket underneath your upper back. You may keep your legs bent or you may extend them, letting your feet flop open to the sides like a fish's tail. Be certain that you don't have pressure on your head. You can use your upper arms to help support you. Stay here as long as you are comfortable. First try to start with five deep inhale/exhale cycles. Then, see where it goes from there.

To Come Out of the Pose

Increase the pressure on your arms and carefully tip your chin to your chest as you lift up your head. Roll to one side and extract the prop that was behind your back. Lie back down on the mat, pause, and notice how you are feeling.

With pen in hand, go to your notebook and record your impressions. These can be at the energetic, physical, emotional, intellectual, and bliss levels. Note how your throat and neck feel. Do you feel able to speak about how you truly feel? Do you feel grounded enough to hold space for another person's truth?

"When the yogini is firmly established in truthfulness, she attains the fruits of actions without acting."
SUTRA 2.36

"The universal vows are non-violence, truthfulness, non-stealing, moderation, and non-greed."
SUTRA 2.30

"The absence of ignorance ends the conjunction of the Seer (Parusha) and the Seen (Prakriti). This is the liberation of the Seer."
SUTRA 2.25

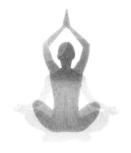

Chapter Nine

MODIFY AND ENHANCE

— STEP NINE —

We made direct amends to such people wherever possible,
except when to do so would injure them or others.

Step Nine required both courage and humility. I had to lose all of my
arrogance and be brave enough to move forward, even when I felt fear
or shame. Half of me wanted to rush through and complete this step
and get it over with. The other half wanted to delay the step as long as
possible. Almost more than any other step, I found I needed to consult
with my sponsor time and again.

I experience what I call emotional blackouts. When I am
overwhelmed with feelings of any kind, good or bad, the adrenaline
rushes through me. While it appears to others that I am present, and
while I do behave normally, my brain doesn't log my actions into long-
term memory. I forget what others have said and how I have responded.
This was a huge problem for me as I approached Step Nine. I was afraid
my emotional state would cause me to forget what was being said. I

was worried that I would forget what we talked about and how we had concluded things when making verbal amends. The fear was real, embedded in fact. It indeed happened once or twice when I took this step in early recovery. I know I had contacted people, but I had not prepared properly, had rushed into things, and then had no memory about what had transpired. It was not the best way to approach the step. Yet that did not stop me from continuing.

The *Twelve and Twelve* indicates that Step Nine is evidence of our willingness to embark on a new phase of life—one in which we are willing to take responsibility for our actions. I needed to be stable, grounded, and firm in my recovery. I needed to feel assured that I was not endangering my recovery by speaking, writing, or meeting with individuals on my list. I needed also to be certain of making apologies or amends from a genuine place. Pleasing others or pleasing my sponsor had no place here. I had to be willing to state my side of the issue, without rationalizing, defending, or justifying my actions.

In addition, I had to be circumspect in observing the warning that we were not to "injure them or others." There were things I had done that I could only mention to my sponsor and, in my case, my therapist, as telling the people involved would have not been beneficial to any party. There were not many of these, but I did need to separate those from the other situations, people, and issues on my list. For these unique cases, there would only be a resolution to never repeat that type of behavior. I could not unburden myself to the people directly; I just had to lead a moral life. I would change my actions to match my ethics and new way of living.

There were people on my list with whom I had started my amends the moment I began my road to recovery. Sobering up was the apology they needed. Mom, Dad, my siblings, and other relations all got to be with a more authentic me—one who wasn't hung over or racing to get away to get loaded. I did actually apologize to them. They didn't want anything else from me; they only wanted me to be well.

It turned out that apologizing was all I needed to do for most people. In other cases, I needed to make further amends: financial repayment, direct apology, and asking what else I could do to make things right.

I may not even have been aware of additional harms I had done, and I needed to give people space to tell me. I had to be brave enough to listen to their anger or disappointment. Also, there were people on my list to whom I could give only partial amends. I wanted to let my friends know I was sorry I had been so unreliable, messy, and selfish. Other things I could not say, as it would have hurt them more, because disloyalty and unfaithfulness involve other people in the apology who may themselves be hurt.

Making Step Nine amends is not done to make us feel better, or to get something off our chest, but to unburden the other person from needing to harbor an unspoken difficulty between us. Once again, no justification is necessary. Listening to the other person's response is of utmost importance.

Some people had passed away, so I couldn't tell them directly what I wanted to say, nor could I rely on a living amends to make things right, as they had no chance to talk to me or tell me their wishes. I created a ritual to coalesce my confession and plans for reparation. I wanted a way to complete the cycle of my past behaviors and document the beginning of my new, more responsible self. This ritual gave me a sense of completeness. I was also able to commit to new behavior with this ceremonial process.

I discovered that I was unable to connect with some people. They had moved away, and some had changed their names, or I had known them only through nicknames and street names. There are numerous ways to track down people now, but when I first did Step Nine there was no internet—we had only the white pages book and calling 4-1-1 operators. For these people, too, I had to find some kind of conclusion, a resolution to my previous behavior, as they were on the list for a reason, and I needed a way to heal the energy between us. My ritual worked in this situation, too.

In my first years of recovery, when initially guided through the steps, I was not practicing yoga. I didn't have the tools I now have or the skills I have been learning and practicing. I had some good, basic guidance from my sponsor. She helped me to develop a ceremony that would bring release and honor to the absent person. We used a scented candle, a written note, and fire. The candle symbolized the absent person, bringing light to the dark parts of our relationship; the flickering flame represented transformation. The note needed to be specific, honest, and complete. I wrote with the candle lit and then safely burned the note so the smoke would dissipate into the atmosphere, in the hope it would reach the essence of the person to whom I was writing. This was sufficient. It was a special way to show respect for the person I was addressing.

Niyamas and Step Nine

Discipline is the principle associated with Step Nine. It is one thing to think about making amends and apologizing, but it is quite another to take action, make contact, set a meeting, prepare yourself, share, and listen. It can make your heart race and feel as if it is stopping at the same time. Be brave. Tapas means "discipline," but it also means "transformation." Step Nine can be truly transformative. It changed me from a woman who was living in dark, tamasic energy and stagnating in the sins of the past to one who is living a more sattvic and harmonious life, finding freedom from her past behaviors. And according to Reverend Jaganath Carrera:

> We need that kind of one-pointed perseverance to overcome obstacles, and pierce the veneer of ignorance. We should never give up. Many people quit when they are on the brink of success. Determination always pays off. Ants, daily walking the same path across a stone wall, will wear a groove in it one day. Likewise, our practices will eventually eradicate ignorance.

Yamas and Step Nine

We want neither to mistreat ourselves nor to put others in danger of harm. We cannot imperil others by coming clean about something. We must find another way to put things right. If it is a financial issue, then repaying anonymously may be sufficient. If it involved others, such as a situation of adultery, it wouldn't be useful to apologize to the other parties. Being honorable and true is the amends. Apologizing over and over again to someone could be interpreted as us seeing something wrong in that person as a result of what we had done to him or her.

This occurred with my child. In later recovery—years after I had sobered up and made my initial apology to my daughter—I continued to apologize to her for having been a negligent mom. She is a terrific mother, and my comment was meant to say, "How did you get to be such a good mom—having me as a mother?" The apology actually kept the focus on me and my feelings rather than on her. Additionally, it sounded to her as though I was comparing our parenting. She was crushed. I was overwhelmed with grief about her pain. I returned to my therapist, who helped me to understand that repeated apologies could be harmful, and continuing to make them was keeping the conversation centered on me rather than her. My daughter is a good mom, period—no reason to remind or compare.

Non-harming includes right speech. When we make amends, we need to frame our comments about our side of the street. It needs to be truthful, kind, timely, and useful.

Kleshas and Step Nine

In our process of working the steps, our ego needs to be checked at the door. Rather than feeling oversized or undersized, I tried to come from a place of being right-sized, a place of grounded certainty, as I prepared for in Step Nine. I approached the conversations without the need to be forgiven, understood, or absolved. I needed to know to the core of my being that I was not a bad person. I had done bad, unfortunate, clumsy, inconsiderate things. I did not have to identify myself by them, but I needed to take responsibility for them. Those are two entirely different things.

The yogic concept of the ego guides us into separating our true nature from what we do or feel. Our true nature is eternal; our actions are temporary. We can change our actions, though we cannot alter our true inner being.

Koshas and Step Nine

We need to learn how to bring our whole self together when making amends and consciously align all the parts of ourselves before making apologies, to avoid acting on impulse. We must get centered to be certain we know how and why we are reaching out.

I clearly remember one of my first amends-making situations. I was in my first eighteen months of recovery and was dead-set on making this amends—I needed to apologize to this man right away. I had not talked it through with my sponsor, and had barely completed my Eighth Step with her. I just knew I had to call him and speak with him. I hadn't planned what I would say, so I was nervous, ungrounded, shaky, and approaching an emotional blackout with short breath, buzzing ears, and my thoughts jumping around.

I found his number and called, introduced myself, and explained in an unclear way what I was doing. I hadn't accounted for the time difference—it was much later where he lived, and thus not a convenient time to have called him. My energy, body, feelings, intellect, and spiritual awareness were all disconnected. I cried, blubbered, and said I was sorry, giving no specifics or the meat of the apology. I just cried, and he said it was okay—as far as I can remember—and I abruptly hung up. I lost my recollection of what I wanted to say, and after the call, I didn't remember what he had said. It was too soon and disorganized, although heartfelt, and not useful. The timing was off due to my haste—my ego was driving the train; my energy level was too high—and I would eventually need to make amends again.

Samskara and Step Nine

Yoga poses and meditation are some of the ways I make amends to myself. The samskara, or the habits of the mind, take time to be reset and refreshed, channeled in a different, more healthful way. That takes dedication. In active addiction and codependency, I was creating mental impressions based on my need for instant gratification, a sense of pleasure without effort, and a need for affirmations and approval from others in order to feel worthy and have self-esteem. When I started recovery, my senses of pleasure, approval, and feeling complete and happy had to come from somewhere other than drugs. I transferred this to people pleasing, which wasn't healthy, and it took another fellowship to address and heal this. I found out that I had to look inside myself. This became the form of the amends.

In making amends to myself, I started by using kinder words when referring to myself. I began to find ways to pause, reflect, and choose rather than run pell-mell into options and opportunities, and even activities in the day. I learned to take time for myself. It wasn't comfortable, but it was necessary.

Putting It All Together

In later recovery, I have expanded my process of making these internal, self-directed amends. I find gratitude and acceptance in forming contentment. I reach for my higher power to remain connected to my higher self. I practice yoga and meditation to release the hold my mind habits have on me and to make space for a more positive, healthy mind-set and point of view. I practice all yamas and niyamas and find many ways of caring for myself and my health, using all levels of my koshas and chakras. I am not perfect, but I make progress.

When amends need to be made, get organized, speak with your sponsor, and take time to meditate. Your intent is to make apologies true, honorable, and timely. Your amends and the changes you bring to relationships and your life come from a grounded, balanced person looking to bring harmony to his or her life.

Pose for Step Nine: Standing Mountain

To prepare for direct or indirect amends, or any apology, you must prepare yourself. Having already done a lot of work to determine the how, what, and why of your past unpleasant behaviors, you can call on the best of yourself to meet the other party, or parties, with humility and strength. Standing mountain is the pose that will give you the gift of standing on your own two feet as you address others.

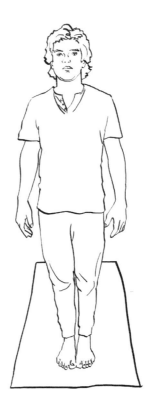

To Come Into the Pose

Standing mountain is a pose of immense strength, balance, and integration. It is fundamental—but like recovery, it is simple but not easy. It is best to practice with bare feet. From any standing position, bring your feet under your hipbones, with the inner or outer edges parallel to one another. Take some time to adjust your feet; move around until the tops of your feet line up under the front bump of your hipbones.

Pay attention to the sensations of your soles on the floor, gaining an awareness of balance. Notice the distribution of your weight by noting the pressure on the soles of your feet. Experiment with rocking forward and back and side to side, then come to stillness with your weight distributed between the balls of your big toe and little toe and the center of the back of your heel. Bring awareness to your legs, engaging the muscles around your lower legs, knees, and thighs.

Engage your stomach and gluteus muscles, gaining length in your waist by drawing up on your spine with the back of your head. Draw your lower front ribs together and back toward your spine. Still breathing, drop your shoulder blades onto your back, align the bottom of your chin with the ground, and reach the top of your head upward. With arms hanging by your sides, use your eyes to gaze softly in front of you.

Breathe again and see how you feel. Be aware of your feet being grounded, your body feeling integrated, and your head balancing in dignity.

To Get Out of the Pose

Step off the mat. Remain integrated and centered. Now, you can face life on life's terms and address your amends with courage and humility. The practice here is to center yourself each time you prepare to make amends. Now would be a good time to write about your ability to be grounded and integrated as you make your amends. Reflect on this step and make some notes about tools that would be helpful to you.

"Austerities destroy impurities and,
with the resulting perfection in the mind,
body, and sense organs,
physical and mental powers awaken."

SUTRA 2.43

"Once attaining the utmost purity of nirvicara,
there is the dawning of the spiritual light,
peace and luminosity of the true self."

SUTRA 1.47

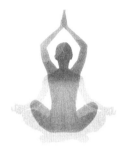

Chapter Ten

DAILY PRACTICES

— STEP TEN —

We continued to take personal inventory and
when we were wrong promptly admitted it.

Step Ten offers a convention for keeping our side of the street clean on an ongoing basis. It is a process for keeping our house in order and releasing quarrelsome thoughts and recollections, plus there's a good chance of being able to rest well each night. Committing to make a regular review of our actions and attitudes gives us a chance to avoid accumulating a new compendium of harsh and unspoken words, unlovely behavior, and selfishness. Working this step also gives us the opportunity to reflect on areas in which we have made progress, practiced good habits, and upheld self-esteem, ethics, and values. As such, Step Ten is both a reflection and an action step.

Newcomers often talk about jumping to Step Ten before completing the previous nine: moving right into evaluating each day and hoping not to add to the wreckage of the past. Already eager to try their recovery wings and wanting to move into healthy ways of treating themselves and others, they start a daily review or a spot-check inventory, as described in the *Twelve Steps and Twelve Traditions*. As the result of their newfound way of being—ceasing the lying, the cheating, and other harmful behaviors—newcomers are learning to respond to their feelings inside when they do something outside. This is an important aspect of getting clean, knowing how you feel and noting it. There is nothing wrong with doing Step Ten in this way early on.

For those of us who have done all the steps, sometimes multiple times, the Tenth Step may feel automatic. Some people have adopted this easily as a daily practice. Others, however, may do it only when the need arises, when something of great note has occurred. This less-than-regular review may have come about due to ennui, laziness, or a sense of "I've got this," the illusion that we do not need to review our behavior because it is all beyond reproach.

Resting on our laurels and letting go of a regular and disciplined practice of the Tenth Step can be dangerous. We may be in that field of boredom with our program, finding no life in our life. We may have become complacent in our assumption that we already know how to act and respond, all the time. I certainly thought so. I assumed I was well. When I hit my bleak patch in the "teenage years" of my recovery, I was happy with my job, my relationships, and my financial security. I was still going to meetings, but I had stopped some of my regular practices such as a regular tenth-step inventory. This deprived me of two things: noticing when I behaved badly, and noticing when I behaved well.

I listened to people talk about the Tenth Step at meetings. I heard some old-timers say they didn't do this daily, and others said they didn't do it on a regular basis. While I certainly apologized immediately when I had spoken harshly or been rude *when I realized it,* I also had stopped making time for a daily reflection on my choices and actions. That period coincided with when I careened into my recovery bottom. This doesn't mean that lacking a daily Tenth Step will lead to relapse; it means only that my personal recovery practices began to slide away. It was a sign. I found that along with getting back in touch with my emotions and releasing trauma through the physical practice of yoga, I needed to return to the discipline of the basics of recovery. I encourage you to do this, too; for at least thirty days, make this a daily practice and see what happens.

When working with my sponsees—many of whom have double-digit sobriety—I find that when we take a moment to contemplate the activities of the day, we tend to see the challenges and the behaviors we wish we avoided rather than those that we did well. It is natural to look at what we can improve. There is value in noticing when we have behaved in a manner that is not in accordance with our new freedom and happiness. Just as a captain on a ship knows the direction of the next port, he or she must adjust to the changing tides, winds, and rate of speed. So we, too, keep monitoring our behavior to see if we can move toward who we want to be and know whether our actions and thoughts will get us there.

Unfortunately, we often stop with the negative. The majority of the people I work with, those to whom I speak with, and those whom I write to stop at the consideration of the adverse and unfavorable. A lot of time is spent looking at the errors, the mistakes, and the negative language, attitude, or behavior. This is informative, and the prior steps can help provide a window to what is going on, but again, it is only part of the step. Our inventory needs to include the useful items, the behaviors that we are working and improving on, the fact we are *doing* the step, and the "thank you, higher power" gratitude that we can take into account in this process each day.

Niyamas and Step Ten

I have found using the observances, the niyamas, as a guide for practicing Step Ten as a way to capture my day thoughtfully.

Cleanliness

Analyzing not only what one says but also how one thinks and acts can be viewed through the lens of the niyama of cleanliness. "What we think we become" is a phrase attributed to the Buddha, and it is the basis of some forms of modern psychology. When we monitor our thoughts, we can discern how these manifest in feelings, reactions, and behavior. If we use a regular check-in to get in touch with how we are thinking during Step Ten, we will have more positives than negatives in our inventory.

Discipline

The quality of discipline is one I practice each day while I take Step Ten. Even when I am tired, even when I think there is nothing to review, even when I would rather just do it in the morning, I pause and practice my Tenth Step. If I don't, I will then owe an amends to myself; the lazy part of me was not caring for the part of me that wants to get well, be well, and do well.

Yamas, Kleshas, and Step Ten

Honesty, or non-lying, plays a large role when I review my day. It keeps my interactions the right size. Avoiding both overstating and understating the occurrences in the day helps me remain humble in a way that addresses both the difficult and the beneficial.

A challenge when reviewing the day can also be our attachment to the outcome of any of our interchanges with others. We can perseverate, going over events and reminding ourselves of opinions, hopes, and assumptions. We must let go of this grasping, and the klesha of avoidance, as we review the day. This is an inventory, not a plenary session, wherein we decide how we are going to approach the situations for an outcome that we desire. It is only a review of how we have been and what we may need to repair.

In order to avoid needing to apologize for the same thing over and over, and to promote the ability to find value and virtue in our Step Ten, we need to dig deep to find out why we had that misstep or how we had come to make that good choice.

Chakras and Step Ten

We can use the chakras to guide us as we make a list of how our day has gone.

Root Chakra

Starting with the root chakra, we can begin to review what we have done before in the previous steps. What has your sense of security, both financial and personal, been? How has your connection with family been? Do you feel grounded, like you have a right to be here on this planet, rather than being apologetic for your existence? Have any challenges in these areas affected how you act?

Sacral Chakra

Proceeding to an evaluation of the sacral chakra, we can ask ourselves how our relationship with a loved one has been. Have you been expressing intimacy and connection in a healthy way? Have you experienced a free-flowing energy of creativity? Have you been flirtatious or inappropriately bawdy in your speech or actions? Did your day offer any challenges in these areas?

Solar Plexus Chakra

What is your level of self-compassion and self-esteem? Were you able to express yourself with self-confidence? If our behavior or thoughts leaned toward the self-critical or fear of rejection, then the solar plexus chakra may be out of balance.

Heart Chakra

If we are open and filled with joy, love, and compassion, then the heart chakra is in balance, and we have positive attributes to include in our inventory. If it is out of balance or underenergized, we may feel jealous, possessive, and tender around the issue of abandonment. This may impact our reactions and responses to others in a negative way, which is good information to discover during our inventory.

Throat Chakra

If we are feeling out of control or experiencing an inability to express ourselves and speak up, our throat chakra may be blocked. The desire to be heard may come out sideways: being overcontrolling or vocal in an unrelated area. For example, we may have transformed frustrations with a boss, coworker, or other person into sharp speech with a loved one who is innocent of the aggravation. However, we should also note in our inventory when we are able to speak freely, expressing ourselves fully in comfort and compassion. This is good information to build on.

Third Eye Chakra

If we are stuck in our inventory, unable to calm down or commit to taking it, our third eye chakra may be blocked. We may be moody, unsettled, or dismissive of others at meetings or of the meetings entirely. Our ability to look inward may be hampered. Or today we get it: the big picture is revealed, and we are able to connect wholeheartedly with our self and others. We are open to receiving wisdom and trusting our own insight.

How did this come about? Did you have a great sleep? Did you eat well today? Did you experience a nice balance of personal time and time with others? Did you adhere to a series of promised activities throughout the day—meditation, reading, meetings, connections, duties, and downtime? Taking the time to notice this is important so that you can refer to it in the future.

Crown Chakra

Our crown chakra is balanced when we feel in balance, connected to our higher power, and able to be in the moment, at least for several moments at a time. If we are out of balance, we may feel depressed, ultrasensitive to sensory input, rigid, or confused, and we may reach back into old prejudices or other forms of separation and alienation. Connection both outwardly to our higher power and deep inside to our true self can help balance and revitalize the crown chakra.

Gunas and Step Ten

I value the qualities of being steadfast as well as the qualities of adaptability and change, which can be a balancing act. When evaluating my day, I look at times when I was firm when being flexible would have been wiser, and I take account of when I held fast to my boundaries with good results in self-care and self-respect. There are also situations where the benefit would have been the reverse: holding firm when I could have been accommodating and being more malleable when I was inflexible.

This is the dance between harmony and activity: sattva and rajas. When I withdraw and become pouty in words or actions, I am being tamasic. At the end of the day, using the yogic words can help me reflect on where I was on the continuum of the three gunas and gain some insight into what was useful and what I would do another way next time. The qualities I honor have qualities themselves.

Koshas and Step Ten

My end-of-day inventory includes taking a quiet moment, a personal check-in, to evaluate my connection with my five koshas. I gauge my energetic reserves and the status of my physical, mental, and wisdom layers, and I reconnect with my higher power. This is another way I can check my assets and liabilities or how I utilize my vitality over the course of the day.

If we are blocked or depleted, out of touch or drained, it is a sign that we met some portion of our day ill-prepared. We most likely allowed one of our shortcomings to reemerge, as we possibly felt hungry, angry, lonely, or tired. We need to evaluate which event or situation caused this or suffered as the result of our drained and weakened state. If we are in touch with all layers, and they are dynamically interconnected, then this has been a great day. We most likely have faced the day with an integrated sense of self and have more on the asset side of our inventory.

Putting It All Together

Step Ten is so delicious; it offers a way to stay connected to our ethics and our values. It is a way to remind us not to step too far off the beam, to stay in the narrower path on the amazing highway of recovery. Just as newcomers jump ahead to make a daily assessment of how their actions measure up with their newfound focus on recovery, it is important, even vital, that we in longer-term recovery approach this step with this same enthusiasm.

Remain disciplined in doing this daily inventory. Use your kit of spiritual tools and add to them the structure of the yogic way to assess and address your assets and liabilities, directed toward others and yourself. You are a beloved child of the universe and deserve the attention from doing Step Ten and the focus of receiving the benefits of it as well.

Pose for Step Ten: Swinging the Torso from Side to Side

Taking inventory happens all the time, although you may choose a regular time of day to do a thorough job of it. After practicing the principles of recovery, you may check in with yourself throughout the day, noting times you handled something with skill and other times you could have used a little more wisdom in your response or action. Your internal monitor is more finely tuned to how you want to be and how you want to behave. However, a regular time to check in is always recommended. You forget both the good and the less than good. In the meantime, you scan yourself and your motives, choices, and interactions. This gentle twisting motion reminds you of this process.

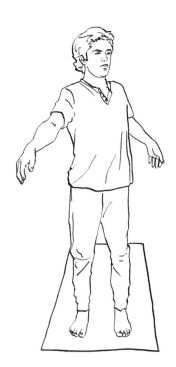

To Come Into the Pose

Stand with your feet hip width apart, in a looser way than mountain pose. Soften your knees so they are not rigid. Begin to twist your body from left to right. Let your arms fling along with this motion, swinging them freely, one in front of the body and one behind. You may even tap your front shoulder and your lower back with your hands as you swing. Keep this up for two minutes. Compare how you feel when you turn your head with each twist to when you keep your face forward. Notice if the pace changes. Notice how you breathe. Do you synchronize the pace with your movement and breath? Just notice. See if you can observe without changing or resisting. You will learn something about yourself.

To Get Out of the Pose

Slow down the movement over the next few breaths, then cease moving completely and stand in stillness. Take your time to just be in the afterglow of that persistent movement. Rest. Write down your reflections on Step Ten and, perhaps, the commitment to practice this step regularly over the next few weeks or months.

"The knowledge gained in that state
is one of wisdom and insight."

SUTRA 1.48

"The ultimate goal of yoga is to always
observe things accurately, and therefore
never act in a way that will make us
regret our actions later."

T. K. V. DESIKACHAR

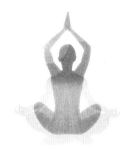

Chapter Eleven
CONNECTION

— STEP ELEVEN —

We sought through prayer and meditation to improve our conscious contact with God *as we understood Him*, praying only for knowledge of His will for us and the power to carry that out.

Prayer and meditation are words that can elicit a sense of calm, serenity, and support—things that we all yearn for. On the other hand, they can also rekindle doubts about spirituality and concerns about our ability to meditate. As with the other steps, there is both hope and challenge in taking Step Eleven.

For years, my active mind and restless body did not make friends with these practices on a consistent basis. My form of prayer was to gasp out for help and mercy when in pain, certainly making genuine appeals for someone when asked. I observed the moment of silence at the beginning of meetings, but a formal practice of prayer and meditation was difficult.

Being overwhelmed with the psychic handcuffs of perfectionism, I was afraid of doing it wrong. My only model for prayer was what I remembered from infrequent church attendance. I went along with it but I felt like a fake in actual practice. It wasn't comfortable then, and was not something that I felt I could do now. The innocent child kneeling at bedside with precious hands clasped before her soft and pouty face was not a pose I wanted to take, or fake. My one heartfelt prayer had been on my first day sober: "God, please help me stop!" After that point, I felt that my prayers were self-serving and not spiritually based. Occasionally they were okay when they were done at a specific request for someone else, but sometimes even this felt shallow. I felt I was giving directions rather than listening.

In my experience, the difficulty has to do with my personal concept of a higher power, which is more in line with a universal spirit. This energy, or being, is equally and evenly within us all and doesn't need my suggestions. Even the recommended prayers from the Big Book do not feel authentic to me. The one exception is the Serenity Prayer—it has a power all its own. I do honor the intention of the other prayers, which allows me to be of maximum service, but that is it. Using the steps and my lust for life helps me find my purpose, and any type of prayer allows me to become all that I can or need to be to fulfill this purpose.

A formalized asking practice I have found comfort in is the Buddhist practice of metta. It is a way to align myself with a wish of well-being for all people. I construct and repeat phrases, or use ones designed by others, to state specific intentions for all beings, including myself. I practice letting go of ill will, resentments, fear, and self-centeredness, and as a result, I am more prepared to be of service to others.

My yoga practice is from the Himalayan Yoga Tradition. This program offers writings on prayer and the practice of going inward. It also teaches that prayer practice is a developmental study. We don't jump into it all at once. We go through deepening stages according to the practices and traditions of our faith journey. The teaching is that prayer can lead us deeper into the core of our being, moving our focus from the external to the internal, the conscious to the subconscious. It is reassuring to me that there are many ways to pray, no one right way, which is a huge relief.

Prayer may not be an issue for you; it may be a part of your practice already. Find and remain with your own path. Your personal relationship with your higher power will guide you to the most dependable and valid way to communicate with her/him/it. Enjoy, practice, and continue to be mindful, paying particular attention to how you feel when you focus in that way and honor it.

Meditation is an important part of the Eleventh Step, yet it often confuses people and gives them pause. What is meditation and how do I do it? Is there a special recovery way? Is there a better way, a right way, or a preferred way? In early recovery, I asked my sponsor to help me meditate. She suggested that I sit quietly and gaze at a candle flame. What I really wanted was for her to sit and show me. Just let me be quiet, be by her side, and watch. Then, I would know what to do, what it would look like, and when I was done. She never offered. I never asked.

Over a decade later, my incessant inability to be still or rein in my mind from its incessant busyness and constant remembering and planning nearly caused me to relapse. The mental activity and disturbances I was experiencing caused me deep emotional unrest. It altered my way of looking at the world, changing what had been an optimistic demeanor into a pessimistic and distrustful one. I was succumbing to negative self-talk and an anxious point of view. I was emotionally and energetically exhausted and ready for a change.

There is a Buddhist proverb that states, "When the student is ready, the teacher will appear." And, I was lucky to find my teacher when I did. A talented and compassionate yoga teacher, she introduced me to breath control and meditation. I sat with her. She showed me a way.

Since then, I have discovered many ways to meditate. I have sat with groups and I have sat alone. I have been in silence and I have followed spoken, guided imagery. I have practiced for as little as two minutes and for as long as a day. Each occasion has its own challenges, and in my steady practice I have discovered that meeting the challenge *is* the practice.

Understanding how yoga develops its approach to meditation can be useful in our recovery. It is a deliberate and multistep process. It starts off slowly. We begin with practicing the basic yamas: non-harming, non-lying, non-stealing, non-excess, and non-attachment. Then, we practice the niyamas such as cleanliness, contentment, discipline, self-study, and surrender. Once we have understood these principles and have begun to apply them in our daily lives, we begin with our mat practice, hatha yoga. The asana practice is complex and can open our awareness to the preferences and fluctuations of the mind and help us move knots of hidden emotions out of our system. After the poses, we move on to the breath practices, known as pranayama. Pratyahara, or the withdrawal of the senses, comes next. In this process, we become aware of our major sense groups and then withdraw from the information we have gathered, letting go of sound, touch, sight, and then conscious thought.

Following these skills, we practice one-point-focused concentration, preparing the mind for its ultimate goal of meditation. This process helps clear the mental landscape, as the steps have done, and prepares the mind to be alone with itself. In other words, we have the presence of mind to find the present in the mind.

Our previous steps have cleared a path to Step Eleven through our inventory, sharing, and atonement for us to arrive at prayer and meditation. The principles of recovery and yoga have prepared us for the practice. We've taken some time to investigate the mercurial nature of the mind and considered the human condition by examining the kleshas, our obstacles. We have explored the influences of energy trapped and energy that is overactive by studying our chakras. We have taken time to evaluate the gunas, the conditions of all things and their impact on our actions, attitudes, and emotions. The body has been prepared for uninterrupted sitting by having stretched, strengthened, balanced, and relaxed. Now we are ready. We are ready to go inside ourselves in an undisturbed way.

By clearing and cleaning the mind and the emotions, we are better prepared to sit with the waves of thought and non-thought that are part of the land of meditation. We are also prepared to accept the reality that change is inherent in all things; nothing is permanent. Unrest is not permanent; calm is not permanent. We discover that being disturbed is part of the practice; the practice is observing and noting our disturbances. Will you respond to the fluctuations of the mind with a gentle ease and know that that is exactly the way it is supposed to be? Or, will you resist and rebel?

Meditation Guidance

Meditation comes in many different forms. You can take your time and check out the various types, such as silent meditation and meditation accompanied by music, nature sounds, or the rhythm of a gong or chime. Meditation may be guided with verbal cues or directed imagery. You can sit in a chair or sit on a cushion or a mat, or you may lie down. It is important to get comfortable but to be in a position that will allow you to remain alert. It is beneficial to practice the same position each day, or each time you meditate, for a length of time. Set an intention to choose one position and meditation style and stick with them for a while. If you choose to sit cross-legged, then make a commitment to that position. If you lean against a wall with your legs outstretched, stay in that pose each time you meditate for the next six or eight times. Give yourself a chance to become accustomed to both the position and the process.

The length of time you choose to meditate may vary day to day. When you first begin, start small—even two minutes will suffice. You may then build up slowly from there to five minutes or maybe half an hour. There is no perfect amount of time and there are no rules; however, the brain itself will soften into the space of non-doing most effectively at the twenty-minute mark. Don't let this number prevent you from dedicating yourself to a regular practice.

When to meditate is also a question that can come up. Often, early-morning meditation is most beneficial. It sets the intention and tone for the day. It can be part of a morning ritual and may be the only time you have for yourself all day long. It can be difficult to scoop twenty minutes or a half hour together for yourself later in the day. Life fills up your time in expected and unexpected ways. That can make it a challenge to find a time and place to find quiet and be calm.

Avoid letting perfect be the enemy of good. If you can't practice in the morning, practice when you can. Set aside five minutes at lunch or take a break in the afternoon or before or after a challenging meeting or presentation. The goal is to practice whenever you want to refresh your intention to *be*. You can also practice again, later in the day, or before you go to sleep. You can't overdo it when it comes meditation, so meditate as often and as long as you need and want to.

The observation of tapas, or discipline, is practiced with this step and with meditation in general. Set an intention to meditate and then honor yourself by keeping that intention. If you oversleep or your day takes off extra early and you don't have ten or twenty minutes for a formal time of meditation, sit on the edge of your bed and breathe mindfully, with attention, for a few minutes. Ten to twelve deep, full, intentional breaths can give you the time to get centered and focused and ready for your day. This also fulfills the commitment you made to yourself, one of the building blocks of self-esteem.

While meditating, we may discover our power to engage in the day, or our purpose, with less effort. When looking for the will of our higher power in guiding our actions and efforts, we need to be silent and listen. There may be no big reveal, no transcendent experience or big arrow pointing to our purpose for the day, but in the quiet, our brain has a chance to unclench the fist of our mind to let the previously unknown rise to the surface. When we sit and meditate, "more will be revealed." This is not because we have a question or are guiding the answer, but because we are not.

There can be a sticky wicket between prayer and meditation, wherein there can be a vibrant semantic discussion about where one leaves off and the other one begins. I will leave that to the theologians and just express my truth: meditation, that space of stillness without a specific prayer verse or memorized passage, is the time that I can listen. In my experience, these are the minutes that align my day and my efforts with those of my higher power.

The Benefits of Meditation

Knowing that we can go out into the world as the best version of ourselves is one of the benefits of meditation. We are retraining the brain to have a more positive view of life. We may learn to pause between thought and action. The part of the brain that determines consequences can become more developed. Here are some other documented results from a consistent meditation practice.

Decrease Stress Response

We learn to sit through discomfort and unpleasant mental activity. Our brain changes structure and rewires itself for more healthful responses to stress. We are better able to remain calm in times of difficulty. We experience an active mind with the practice of doing nothing but sitting and waiting for all the information to come in.

Better Concentration Skills

The preparation for meditation includes the practice of one-pointed concentration. In meditation, we practice moving back time and again to the anchor of the sitting practice, whether it is the breath or a flame or a sound. We develop endurance when it comes to redirection. Meditation is being taught to kids in schools in order to help them with their studies. It helps us concentrate wherever we are, whatever we are doing.

Decreases Anxiety and Depression

With the practice of letting go of the difficult, enticing thoughts of the past and staying in the present, we develop a way to self-soothe. Being in breath-centered focus and fulfilling a commitment to ourselves to sit in meditation, we release anxiety and relieve depression.

Easier Focus on Compassion for Self and Others

Having practice in observing the mind, experiencing where the mind goes and what it does before being called back, is a way to make friends with ourselves and our busy brain. When we call the wandering mind back with words of kindness and compassion, these qualities become stronger and more accessible. Positive responses come more easily with practice.

Increase Health and Happiness

Meditation is part of cancer care, used as treatment for coping with chronic pain, and increases our enjoyment quotient, rewiring the brain for happiness. Certain styles, such as Mindfulness-Based Stress Reduction (MBSR), have documented success not only in reducing stress but also in increasing healing from surgeries and medical issues and creating a positive attitude when facing life in general.

Tolerate the Difficult with Greater Ease

A daily consistent practice can calm the nervous system long beyond the time spent in meditation. The day itself, all day long, is easier to face and manage.

Increase Social Connection and Decrease Loneliness

Whether done alone or in groups, the practice of meditation connects us all. Most formal meditation practices include a moment to acknowledge our connection to all beings, as well as a moment to include them in our wishes for peace, tranquility, and safety. Meditation improves your connection within yourself and to the world.

Putting It All Together

Meditation will help you develop what Emma Seppala calls the "badass brain." We rewire our nervous system and reform our response cycles. We learn how to experience and manage deferred gratification—a huge step in relapse prevention. We do this by using stillness, awareness, and the breath to unite body, mind, and spirit. Meditation also increases cortical mass, the part of the brain we need for decision-making, determining consequences, developing self-control and emotional control, and increasing our ability for self-reflection.

The third eye and crown chakras are invigorated and balanced as we practice internal review, which is the delicious intention of the Eleventh Step: finding quiet to discover how we can bring good into the world at large. We become the best version of ourselves and develop the capability to manifest that in our daily lives.

While I have my challenges with the idea of prayer—a semantic challenge, I believe—I open my heart to the suggestions of the universe as I manage my interior landscape in meditation. My ability to speak and live my truth is increased with periods of silence. I move closer to being useful to others and less self-directed. I discover how to be empowered in my life, through unity and spirituality.

Develop your own "badass brain" with a consistent practice of prayer and meditation. See for yourself the yummy results of a steadier mind, more compassionate heart, and greater ability to be your authentic self with consistency.

Pose for Step Eleven: Seated Position

Seeking greater connection with yourself, one another, and your concept of the universal spirit through prayer and meditation starts with a comfortable body. Look toward finding a position that allows you to be comfortable and remain alert at the same time. This is a time to set an intention, putting forth a prayer and listening to the quiet. There are many types of meditation, and as you can get distracted in the Fourth Step trying to find the best method or tools for that step, you may get distracted in Step Eleven to find a special pillow, candle, or narration to begin your meditation. Avoid all that distraction and just sit down. Try it this way, a simple way, to start.

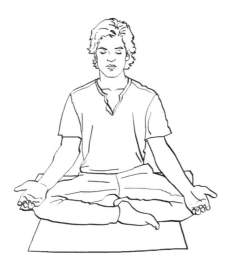

To Come Into the Pose

While meditation *can* be done in a prone position, it is a skillful meditator who can do this without falling asleep. It is best to start in a seated position with or without back support. To prepare yourself for this practice, get comfortable, being certain that you will not get too cool as you sit, and choose a time and place where you are least likely to be interrupted. When sitting cross-legged on the ground, it often helps if the hips are elevated above the level of the knees. You can use a cushion, or several, to sit on and perhaps tuck blankets beneath the knees for support. If sitting cross-legged is not comfortable, you can sit on your heels with your shins on the ground. Again, you can try elevating the hips to decrease pressure on the knees or feet. You can sit on a chair or a sofa. Be comfortable. Lower your gaze or close your eyes. Then begin the method you have chosen; the entry point is often the breath. Set an intention to be in this position for five minutes, or longer if you wish. Use a timer to keep track of the time.

To Get Out of the Pose

When your timer goes off, or when the guiding voice ceases, or when you are ready, bring your hands together and slowly open your eyes. Notice how you feel. Congratulate yourself. Write down your experience, remembering that there is no right or wrong, no good or bad, just a reflection of what you discovered.

"When the yogi is firmly established in non-violence, hostility is abandoned in his presence."

SUTRA 2.35

"For others, the path is faith, energy, mindfulness, meditation, and wisdom."

SUTRA 1.20

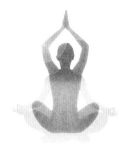

Chapter Twelve

SENTIENCE AND SERVICE

—— STEP TWELVE ——

Having had a spiritual awakening as the result of these steps,
we tried to carry this message to addicts, and to practice
these principles in all our affairs.

In yogic terms, Step Twelve is the step that takes recovery off our yoga mat and out of our meetings and into our life, our community, and the world. We take our inspiration, our ethical practices, and go out into our daily lives carrying the message of hope and recovery, not only in what we say but also in how we behave. These two separate parts and philosophies combine in a powerful way to bring our practice to life.

Initially, when Bill W. and Dr. Bob got together to bring these principles to others, the act of being in recovery was inextricably bound together with the step of carrying the message to others. Staying sober meant getting others sober—all the time, every day. "Wet ones" were actively sought out and, if they were deemed ready, were actively recruited. Once they were enlisted and had a cup of coffee under their belts, they were indoctrinated with three quick steps: accept a higher power, turn your life over, and confess your sins. The process was quick: you came, you came to, and you came to believe all at one time. And the next day, you were out looking for another suffering alcoholic. They lived in the service of the Twelfth Step.

Over the course of time, a more complete and thorough path of steps was drawn between the first three steps and the twelfth. We now do more personal and internal work before we take another person under our wing. This is true of all twelve-step programs: we do our work and then we offer what we have to others. Nevertheless, the spirit of recovery begs to be shared, and I, for one, was eager to share even before I had completed the steps myself. I had tasted hope and wanted others to have some, too.

It is many years later, and my initial enthusiasm has not abated. I love being on this side of my primary diseases—alcoholism, drug addiction, and codependency. I know what addiction is and feels like. My enthusiasm for recovery stems partly from wanting to prevent others from experiencing continued suffering.

Maintaining wise insight and facing life as it comes takes work. The discipline, or tapas, of doing the next right thing, while sounding easy, is not always so. In order to speak truthfully, honestly, and with integrity, I have to keep working the steps. I have to keep up my personal practice if I want to guide and sponsor others. When I have a problem, I bring it to my sponsor; if she isn't available, I move on to connecting with another member of my fellowship. When I find the solution, I share it at a meeting as an example of how it works. I look at areas of my life that are problematic with vigilance, because when I get out of balance my actions, attitudes, and behaviors backslide into pre–steps six- and seven-shortcomings. Yoga keeps me in touch. Yoga has helped guide me to and maintain my spiritual awakening.

The goal of yoga is to help us clear away the noise and illusions of our lives and allow us clearer access to our higher power. What could provide more illusions than the obscuring power of active addiction? Putting the plug in the jug—no matter what form that takes—is a huge step toward preparing ourselves to be in union with our true spirit and higher power. Working the steps, like a full yogic practice, is designed to uncover all the other veils of unconscious and subconscious processes that occlude our spiritual vision. The Twelve Steps are the framework, and yoga can enhance the structure.

A strictly mat yoga practice can be as anemic as restricting myself to the first three steps of recovery. The poses are useful, release stress, and can make one feel wonderful, but to progress to the place where yoga can really change your life, an investigation into the philosophy it offers deepens your experience with the practice.

I worked through the yamas and the niyamas first. I considered them from all sides and applied the steps to them. I applied them to the steps. I investigated kleshas, the obstacles or sufferings, and I noticed how they played out in my steps, particularly in the Fourth Step, the Sixth Step, the Seventh Step, and the Tenth Step. I noticed the influences of a blocked or overactive chakra in the way I experienced and reacted to life. I noticed the qualities of the gunas in the way I felt and perceived others.

With the steps, I had a guide: someone to help me through. I didn't have a guide when using yoga with the steps. I have done a lot of reading and spoken to many people, but I have not had a single unique guide; instead, I have had many. I have used these principles and recommendations with the people I sponsor, and this book was written to share that experience with you.

Doing the steps manifested the spiritual experience I had when I was first able to stop drinking. This spiritual awakening continued when I stopped using drugs completely. I have used the steps on other aspects of my life, such as being the adult child of an alcoholic and addressing the codependent traits that lived with me as the result of that experience. Yoga has made identifying and evolving those behaviors a little easier.

Using the tools of the sutras, the *Bhagavad Gita,* and the instruction of my teachers, my mentors, and the people whom I look up to helped me identify how I respond to limiting thoughts. These illusions of not being enough, feeling overwhelmed, and living life as I imagine *others* want me to are ways to keep me from my true self. In true ironic recovery style, my true self is what I want to recover and come back to. I discovered for myself that the true self is both the source and the goal of my spiritual awakening. I have learned to let this seed self, true self, guide me in how to behave in all of my affairs.

When I discovered that the yogic texts mirrored many principles from twelve-step literature, this "aha moment" launched my unearthing of a stable sense of my true self. The Twelve Steps started the journey; then my yoga study expanded and deepened my ability to identify and investigate my feelings, decisions, and reactions. However, for me as a human being, my awakenings ebb and flow. Each new life circumstance gives me another opportunity to wake up. Each recovered emotional backsliding brings me closer and closer to being my true self.

Now that you have worked the steps in a yogic way, see how you feel each day in all your affairs. With these additional tools, are you able to pause and take stock before you act or speak? Are you able to enjoy your life a little more easily, with less negative internal commentary and a little less comparison to others? I am. I attribute these abilities to the steps *and* to my yoga practice.

Moving the body in asana practice, using my breath in maintaining present-time awareness, and taking time for meditation align me with my intentions for my day and are gifts from both yoga and the steps. But twelve-step practice does not stop with personal awareness; we are offered the healing power of connection by reaching out to others. Service is strongly suggested. Whenever I share my story, whenever I reach out to another person suffering from any addictive disease, I am healing my own samskara of the past, training my brain to recall and reinforce my new way of living.

Dr. Bob and Bill W. were almost frantic in their need to find another alcoholic, one whom they could help. They felt their very lives depended on it. They did not let failure stop them if one drunk was not ready; they tried and tried again. They were undaunted by failure and continued until they eventually found someone who was ready. They found person number three, and at that point they became a meeting. A year later, there were about fifteen of them who had continued to maintain sobriety. They succeeded together as a community.

It is very helpful to meet in groups. Combining recovery and yoga has been a powerful force for change. I have been doing so for several years now, leading meetings in a format designed by Nikki Myers. In my group, it is traditional to apply a yogic concept to the steps of recovery. With a meeting open to anyone recovering from any stage or relationship to addiction, we use the steps of recovery from all behaviors and substances. This modality has been beneficial, allowing us to investigate the steps at a deeper level. The steps also provide a framework with which to investigate and apply the yogic concepts.

Practicing these principles in all my affairs means that I practice the yamas and the niyamas, from non-harming through surrender; use the attributes of hope, discipline, loyalty, and honesty; am true to myself; and avoid inflation or deflation of my ego and false sense of self. I get to move out into the world and be the best I can be. I do this with a number of yogic skills available to me as well as by practicing the steps. I center, I breathe, I become aware of emotions as they're moving around in my body, and I can make peace with them by letting them be. As I notice emotions in my body, I can determine if there is some action I need to take now, or if I need to wait.

I have learned through my fellowship that if there's something wrong with the world through my eyes, it is really wrong with me. The world is the world. Whether I'm looking at it or not, it is what it is. My perspective and my interactions are mine and mine alone. I take into account my feelings about acceptance and remember what I have learned about perception from the yogic perspective of self and not self. I consider the ideas of permanence and impermanence, the "big E" and the "little E" ego, and I realize that if I'm feeling disturbed, then it is likely my impressions and my resistance to taking action on what I perceive.

That does not mean that I will tolerate everything that I see, it does not mean that I give up and turn my back on what I observe and feel, and it does not mean that I need to take what I see and feel and put up with it. It means I see things as they are, make a choice, and take some time to consider before acting. If I am disturbed, is it something within me? Or, am I in a situation that is untenable, with people who are behaving in an unacceptable way? Do I see an injustice and not stand up to it? I need to evaluate the source of the discomfort, then get to work and practice my principles.

Being of Service to Others

As I mentioned earlier, we may start being of service to others from our first day in recovery. This opportunity allows us to become part of the family, the tribe. Addiction is a disease of separation: feeling different, terminally unique, apart, or isolated. When isolated, we become prey to addictive behaviors and cravings of all sorts. Service is important because it helps us connect. Being of use in the group and contributing is a guaranteed way to become part of it rather than separate from it.

Initially, we may have been asked to set up chairs, help with the coffee, greet people at the door, or read as part of the introduction or conclusion literature for a meeting. Our service expands when we share when called on. We have been asked to chair at meetings, sharing our personal experience, strength, and hope.

Doing work at the level of hospitals and institutions or going into jails or treatment centers to share our story is another way that we offer our services. Combining yoga with this outreach work can bring additional important tools to the recovery toolbox.

By midrecovery, we have probably done a lot of service. We have been a meeting secretary a time or two, have held other offices, and have possibly worked in hospitals and institutions, offering experience, strength, and hope to those newly in recovery. We have been a sponsee and we have sponsored others. We have worked toward bringing the recovery principles into our lives as well as having worked with the newcomers.

However, the memory of our first spiritual experience—either the one that brought us to the rooms the first time or the one that finally kept us there—may have faded. The visceral feelings of that critical and life-changing moment may now be relegated not to an oft-told horror story but to one that is no longer fresh and alive or experienced on a visceral level. We may not speak about it often; it may just come up at our recovery anniversary when we recall what it used to be like. It may no longer be an essential part of what it is like now. The immediacy has faded as time has passed. That is the nature of being human. We awaken only to fall asleep again, maybe not so hard, maybe not so deep. But we forget.

In yoga, we practice waking up. We, too, like people in recovery, know that there is something genuine inside ourselves that longs to be discovered and recovered. It may be far, far back in our childhood, before the madness started, but it is there—our true self. How can we maintain a readiness for spiritual awakenings? Remaining open to acceptance about what we have learned about our past will allow us to move through the experiences. With the practices of gratitude, living an ethical life, understanding the techniques, and the values discussed in the previous chapters, we can welcome our inner selves into the present moment.

Some say that twelve-step programs are selfish programs, in that we concentrate first on getting ourselves well. Although this is true, the real mission of recovery is the work we do during our Twelfth Step. The works that we do and services we perform in support of the Twelfth Step are actually to the benefit of all mankind. This is where the humility that we've learned through the other steps comes into play.

When you do good works and turn the benefit of the good works over to your higher power, then the good works are no longer a reflection of you. This is tremendously important. Our Twelve Traditions as well as the steps guide us. They are helpful in keeping our focus on the good of our particular twelve-step group rather than on ourselves. But as I've said, we are human. There are times when we may erroneously elevate ourselves to an expert, acting as though the benefit of the good reflects on how good or important we are. This is incorrect. We must practice pure karma and leave the outcome to a higher power, disengaging ourselves, our egos, from the result.

The idea of karma being selfless service can be a confusing element of sponsorship. I actually benefit from my service; I remain sober. So, the karma is perhaps not the purest karma. I wish and hope that the person I'm working with also will remain clean and sober. I am not, however, in control of that. It is not a reflection on me. If she remains clean and sober and enjoys many years in recovery, that's on her and her higher power. If she goes out again, if she uses or drinks again, that's on her, and it's between her and her higher power. I remain clean and sober; the person I am working with may not. I have to let that go.

While thinking about karma and not karma and who is benefiting from what, we can become confused. Keep it simple. Yoga teaches us to live in reference to our ethics and values rather than looking at the response of others. Avoid looking to please any other ego-focused inputs when you are in service. That will allow your actions to be pure.

A sponsee asked me if she should feel bad about feeling good when she helps another alcoholic. The simple answer is no, but it is really more complex than that. What is the motivation for helping another? Do you keep looking for some specific feeling (attachment or craving), or do you continue to help others because it is the right thing to do? If others thank you, is that okay? Of course. There are two parts of a gift: the giving and the receiving. However, we need to understand that the outcome is the work and the benefit of the other person and his or her higher power, not our efforts. We are merely offering our time and ear. We are making a safe space for the other person to find her- or himself.

Our higher power, the universe, needs us all with our gifts and challenges. Our successes may benefit others in the form of an example, and our challenges may benefit others as we overcome them. Our challenges are also our gifts to others as they, too, may support us with their time, care, and listening.

Putting It All Together

My plateauing in recovery didn't come from ceasing meeting attendance. It didn't come from abandoning my sponsees or losing touch with my sponsor. It came because I had forgotten. I had forgotten the essences of my true self. I had left behind my understanding of the steps, and in particular, Step Twelve.

In my quest to be the best at my job, to be the best wife to my husband, to *do* rather than to be, I had forgotten that I had had a spiritual awakening. I hadn't taken a pause in years, much less time to reflect on what my recovery had done for my life. I had become complacent and, in a way, self-confident, meaning that I was seeing myself as the author of my life—me alone, forgetting my friends, my sponsors, my sponsees, my supportive family, and my higher power. I no longer consulted with them or checked in, seeking input or advice. I had forgotten in all but words my connection with the universal spirit of connectedness. I was accepting my good fortune as my due. This was part of the cause of my near relapse. I had disconnected. Don't let this happen to you. Reaffirm your relationship to your community and to your higher power at a deep level, with daily practice, and you won't be alone anymore.

Take a moment here in quiet meditation to consider your spiritual awakening. Truly, take a few moments and remember your connection with other beings, your higher power, the work you have done, the opportunities offered you, and the wisdom you have discovered through challenges. Look at the self and the not self and reflect on the ego that is the true you versus the ego that is the misunderstanding of self. Only by being the right size can you authentically go out into the world and make manifest the principles you have practiced in the steps and through yoga.

Pose for Step Twelve: Tranquility Pose

You may want a pillow for your head, an eye pillow, a bolster to use beneath your knees, and a blanket to cover you. Step Twelve is a "being" step as well as an "action" step; ultimately, it is an integration step. We conclude the hatha (mat) yoga with *savasana,* or the tranquility pose. This pose is designed to help you cease an active ego and invite you into a self of be-ing. This is the point of the practice at which all the benefits are absorbed into the five layers: energy, physical, emotional/ intellectual, wisdom, and spiritual. The Twelfth Step refers to a deep, abiding spiritual awakening; savasana bakes that right in. Your more integrated and grounded self embodies the wisdom of the practice and the steps, allowing for a more effective assimilation of your values into all your relationships.

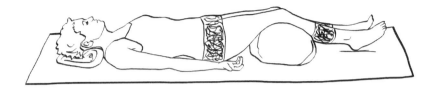

To Come Into the Pose

This is a fully prone back-lying pose. You will want padding beneath you, support for your head and knees, the comforts of a blanket, and perhaps an eye pillow to sooth your eyes. Arranging your props so that you can reach them easily, lie on your back with your heels as wide as or wider than the base of your mat. Your arms should be at your side, with your palms up and away from your body. Some yoga traditions suggest that your upper arms should move away from the torso, so they do not touch the body at all. Find a distance that feels comfortable, one that will not aggravate your shoulders or wrists. Make sure your head rests at a neutral angle with the head fully supported and your face parallel to the ceiling, with neither the neck arched nor the chin tucked. You can choose to remain with your knees bent or straight. You can have a blanket over you or not and an eye pillow on your eyes or not. Try it all and see what gives you comfort. Set a timer for ten minutes. Rest.

To Get Out of the Pose

Begin by moving your fingers and toes. Rock your arms and legs slowly from side to side. Rock your head from side to side. You can reach your arms up onto the ground above your head and stretch your long body. Bring your knees to your chest and hold the backs of your thighs or the backs of your knees. Rock from side to side. Release the right arm over your head and roll to the right. Stay here for a moment.

Bring to mind the purpose of all this work: the clearing, cleansing, and strength, the respect and honor and grace you have brought to your life and the life you share with others. With confidence, know that you have something valuable to share. Say thanks. Push your arms into the ground to come to a seated position. Take a few breaths here before you reenter your life.

Writing after a deep savasana may be difficult, but not impossible. What was your experience in savasana? If you can recall how you felt before the pose and notice how you feel now, you can write a few sentences about that awareness. This is the pause that can refresh.

"For the man who wishes to mature,
the yoga of action is the path;
for the man already mature,
serenity is the path."

THE *BHAGAVAD GITA* 6.3

"That's what you are here for. You are here to serve, here to lift, here to grace, here to give hope and action, here to give the very deep love of your soul to all those who are in need."

YOGI BHAJAN

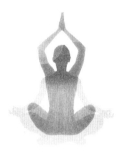

Conclusion

EXPERIENCING A BALANCED LIFE

The book is over; close it, and go on and have a good life. You have worked the steps in the original fashion or you wouldn't be here. And now you have read how to do the steps using some deep, philosophical tools of yoga. Having taken the time and set the intention to improve your conscious contact with a higher power and look inside yourself to figure out how you were standing in your own way, you are now better prepared to participate in your own recovery.

Stalling out in recovery is painful. As in the Peggy Lee song "Is That All There Is?" you may wonder if recovery has become dull. When you are hitting a wall in personal growth, your present circumstances may seem like a poor excuse for the life you imagined. Your job, your family (or lack of family), your opportunities, your achievements, and your losses may seem either overwhelming or bland. You may feel undeserving, as though this life is not yours to keep.

Your life is yours to keep. You can have the successes in your life; you can face the challenges and more. You can connect with others authentically; you can keep your connection to your higher power fresh and strong. You deserve a good, full life, and now you have more tools to tell you how.

Why did I write this book? Why did I take the time to present a process for working the steps using the philosophy of yoga? Why coach you through the sometimes-dry aspects of the mystifying nuances of the ancient wisdom to embellish what the founders of the twelve-step programs have already laid out for us? I set down this study and the work that I have done—by myself and with others—because it is profoundly useful. It gives us a new way to winkle out latent shadows of our past. It gives us new light to shine into the corners of our everyday lives, so they can be more fulfilling and filled with greater ease.

Being human is hard. Being a human and overcoming the disease of addiction—substance or behavior—is really hard. Backsliding is a given; it can be a little and affect us emotionally, or it can be a lot, ending in relapse. In the latter case, it can be dangerous to those of us whose addiction can kill us.

We are a curious lot. We want to know *more* with almost the same passion as when we wanted to have more, eat more, or drink more. Many of us have been questioning the universe and our place in it since we were young. The spiritual solution to our dis-ease has been critical to our healing.

Years after getting clean and sober in my twelve-step program, I plateaued in my development. I also fell into another addiction: work. I have worked with others who have also experienced this malaise. Not everyone turned to work: some turned to food, others to disordered shopping, and several to unhealthy relationships. They didn't relapse in their original addiction but found another form that took them out of balance and disconnected them from their spiritual core. It happened to them, it happened to me, and it may have happened to you.

These new tools you have read about offer the yogic ideals in a western way with a recovery focus. Yoga breaks the sufferings of the human condition down in one way, and the books associated with the many twelve-step programs walk us through the difficult fields of recovery.

I have been working with people who are many years into recovery, and they love their twelve-step groups. They have never stopped attending, but they have hit a dry spell in their personal growth. Intellectually, they have the steps down, know what they are about, and have worked them with both their sponsors and their sponsees—many times and in many ways. And, they feel stuck. Using all forms of yoga has enlivened their recovery and rekindled their enthusiasm for it. Revisiting old behaviors with a new perspective is useful, and going through the beloved and familiar steps with the yoga view invigorated their recovery. Doing mat yoga releases trapped emotions, and using the breath practices gives them new control over how their feelings express themselves. Keeping the old and trying the new can save your life.

Yoga does two things: it gets the body to make peace with the mind and the mind to make peace with the body. As it achieves this, as a practice and not a goal, the wisdom and practicality of the steps are both complemented and reinforced.

I have incorporated the concepts from yoga—the kleshas, the koshas, the gunas, the chakras, the yamas, and the niyamas—into my yoga classes wherever I have taught. I include them when I hold Yoga of 12 Step Recovery (Y12SR) classes. I include them in my meetings with sponsees, either overtly or in an oblique way.

The model of yoga improves and broadens the discussion of our spirituality. Some people are put off by the overwhelming Christian overtones in the literature. They feel separate, as if they don't belong. Even when the books state that it is our higher power—one of our own understanding—it is apparent they are referring to a monotheistic religion. Yoga includes that concept and offers a more universal spiritual connection as well. The language is more neutral.

Using the amazing process of the Twelve Steps, cultivated from Bill W. and Dr. Bob's experience with the Oxford Group, we have been offered an amazing life in recovery. By adding yoga, we can increase our awareness of the steps and not supplant the traditional process.

This book contains more yoga than what we traditionally present in yoga classes. You may have picked this book up thinking that there were poses for each step and a breath practice for the promises. You have been brave and tenacious. You have made it all the way through.

My hope is that you are finding new freedom and happiness. The vicissitudes of life are not removed; your ability to handle them has increased. The ability to identify them as they come up, the skill to note them, the courage to sit with them, and the willingness to do what needs to be done and then to let go has increased. You cannot stop pain, aging, illness, and death, but you are better prepared to understand them.

I thought that when I recovered, all would be well. I also thought that if I ate right, slept right, and went to meetings, life would become easier. In fact, it did not. It became *livelier* because I no longer had the insulation of my intoxication. I could no longer hold onto that illusion. My life, in fact, was not good in any sense during my active addiction. There was the delusion that it would be fine, but it was not. Then, I thought that if I sobered up, all would be well, but it was not. However, being sober let me make better choices, follow plans, handle disappointments, and face life on life's terms.

My disease started before I drank, before I used, as with many of us who have suffered from what I call societal karmic addiction behaviors. My grandparents had challenges growing up that caused them to place some maladaptive behaviors on my parents, who then imparted their version of dysfunctional parenting to me. My mom's parents were emotionally cold and secretive about my grandfather's drinking. They alternated between being welcoming and being reserved and rule oriented. We would visit and sometimes we were included in the activities—the regular grandma cooking and eating fun in the kitchen. The next time we visited, we were cautioned to sit politely on the couches and be still. We never knew which it would be.

My mom struggled with being emotionally available, and retreated often into silence. She would vacillate between being maudlin and inappropriately confiding in us about her difficulties with my dad. Other times, she was wicked strict, and we were punished for behaviors that had been permitted just hours ago. She would also retreat into depressed silence and inactivity, and that terrified us most of all. I became the same with my kids. I was the fun-loving, anything-goes parent. Other times, I would be the rules-setting demagogue I thought represented true parenting. Of course this was at its worst when I was drinking, just as it was for my mom. When I stopped drinking, I had to learn how to parent, but my internal landscape was still designed by my childhood experiences. I had to get help and tools to work on that.

These difficulties are the human condition. Yoga sees the influence of generational stories on each of us. These processes, many of which I explain in this book, were categorized. We can unravel the past and make choices about the future when we move and grow closer to our awakened spiritual self.

You already value your recovery. You read this book to see what other goodness you can squeeze out of your life experiences, what pain you can let go of, and what changes you can make. You have worked the steps through at least once, and probably numerous times. You may have worked them on more than one affliction. You may have used them in one or more aspects of relationships and intimacy. And, you may still find discomfort in your life—a part of the human condition. As documented by the sages and told to us through the ages, we have emotions and self-will. It is up to us to find the tools to help us grow. I hope this path is one of your tools.

"Practice, practice and all is coming."
SRI K. PATTABHI JOIS

OTHER BOOKS BY KYCZY HAWK

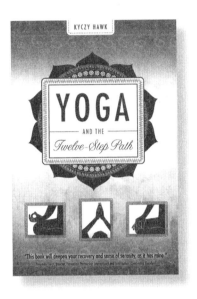

Yoga and the Twelve-Step Path

A blending of principles and disciplines to enhance
and illuminate your Eleventh-Step experience.

PAPERBACK:	978-1-936290-80-2
DIGITAL:	978-1-936290-88-8

Available Spring 2018

Yogic Tools for Recovery Workbook

An active way to extend and strengthen your
yogic investigation of the Twelve Steps.

PAPERBACK:	978-1-942094-63-0
DIGITAL:	978-1-942094-64-7